MEDICAL MATHEMATICS AND DOSAGE CALCULATIONS

D1435150

FOR VETERINARY PROFESSIONALS

MEDICAL MATHEMATICS AND DOSAGE CALCULATIONS

FOR VETERINARY PROFESSIONALS

ROBERT BILL

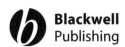

Blackwell
Publishing

Dr. Robert (Pete) Bill, DVM, PhD, is an associate professor of veterinary pharmacology and the assistant to the director of the Veterinary Technology Program at Purdue University School of Veterinary Medicine at West Lafayette, Indiana.

cover and book design: Justin Eccles

Blackwell Publishing Professional
2121 State Avenue, Ames, Iowa 50014

Orders:	1-800-862-6657
Office:	1-515-292-0140
Fax:	1-515-292-3348
Web site:	www.blackwellprofessional.com

Authorization to photocopy items for internal or personal use, or the internal or personal use of specific clients, is granted by Blackwell Publishing, provided that the base fee of $.10 per copy is paid directly to the Copyright Clearance Center, 222 Rosewood Drive, Danvers, MA 01923. For those organizations that have been granted a photocopy license by CCC, a separate system of payments has been arranged. The fee code for users of the Transactional Reporting Service is 0-8138-2099-5/2000 $.10.

Printed on acid-free paper in the United States of America

Library of Congress Cataloging-in-Publication Data

Bill, Robert
    Medical mathematics and dosage calculations for
veterinary professionals / Robert Bill.
        p.   cm.
    ISBN 0-8138-2099-5 (alk. paper)
    1. Veterinary drugs—Dosage—Handbooks, manuals,
etc. 2. Veterinary medicine—Mathematics—Handbooks,
manuals, etc. I. Title.

SF919 .B55 2000
636.089'514—dc21   00-033438

The last digit is the print number: 9 8 7 6 5 4 3

CONTENTS

CHAPTER 1
SELF-ASSESSMENT   3

Self-Assessment Exercise   4
Self-Assessment Exercise Answers   14

CHAPTER 2
DECIMAL NUMBERS   25

SECTION I
THE BASICS OF DECIMAL NUMBERS   25

Relative Values   25
Reading Decimal Numbers Aloud   26
The Rules for Zero in Decimal Numbers   27
Scientific Notation for Decimal Numbers   29
Section I Practice Problems   32

SECTION II
ADDITION AND SUBTRACTION OF
DECIMAL NUMBERS   33

Tips for Adding and Subtracting Decimals   33
Section II Practice Problems   35

SECTION III
MULTIPLICATION OF
DECIMAL NUMBERS   36

Section III Practice Problems   38

SECTION IV
DIVISION OF DECIMAL NUMBERS 39

  Section IV Practice Problems 42

SECTION V
ROUNDING OF DECIMAL NUMBERS 43

  Section V Practice Problems 45
  Answers for Practice Problems 46
  Chapter 2 Problems 47

CHAPTER 3
FRACTIONS 51

SECTION I FRACTION BASICS
AND SIMPLIFYING FRACTIONS 51

Numerators and Denominators 51
Improper Fractions, Proper Fractions,
  and Mixed Numbers 54
Finding Equivalent Fractions 56
Simplifying or Reducing Fractions 58
  Section I Practice Problems 60

SECTION II
ADDITION AND SUBTRACTION
OF FRACTIONS 60

Adding Fractions 60
Finding the Common Denominator
  for More Complex Fractions 62
Subtraction of Fractions 64

Addition of Mixed Numbers   65
Subtraction of Mixed Numbers   67
  Section II Practice Problems   69

SECTION III
MULTIPLICATION OF FRACTIONS   70

Multiplication of Improper Fractions   71
Multiplication of Whole Numbers
    and Fractions   72
Multiplication of Mixed Numbers   72
A Shortcut for Multiplying Fractions   72
  Section III Practice Problems   75

SECTION IV
DIVISION OF FRACTIONS   76

The Reciprocal   76
Division of Fractions   77
Division of Mixed Numbers   78
  Section IV Practice Problems   79

SECTION V
CONVERSION OF FRACTIONS
TO DECIMALS   80

  Section V Practice Problems   82

SECTION VI
CONVERSION OF DECIMALS
TO FRACTIONS   82

Rounding Fractions   84
Section VI Practice Problems   86
Answers for Practice Problems   87
Chapter 3 Problems   90

CHAPTER 4
PERCENTAGES   95

SECTION I
DEFINITION AND USE
OF PERCENTAGES   95

Conversion of Percentages to Fractions   96
Conversion of Percentages to Decimals   97
Conversion of Fractions to Percentages   98
Section I Practice Problems   98

SECTION II
USING PERCENTAGES TO SOLVE
PROBLEMS   100

Finding the Percentage of a Whole   101
Subtracting or Adding the Percentage
    of the Whole   104
Determining Percentages Represented by
    the Fractional Component   105
Section II Practice Problems   107
Answers for Practice Problems   108
Chapter 4 Problems   109

CHAPTER 5
SOLVING FOR THE
UNKNOWN VALUE X   111

SECTION I
FINDING THE VALUE OF
THE UNKNOWN X IN ADDITION
AND SUBTRACTION   112

Analyzing the Problem and Setting
    Up the Equation   112
Moving the Values from One Side of
    the Equation to the Other   114
Moving Negative Numbers of
    Unknown X in Subtraction   117
Section I Practice Problems   121

SECTION II
FINDING THE VALUE OF
UNKNOWN X IN MULTIPLICATION
AND DIVISION   122

Finding the Unknown X in a
    Multiplication Problem   123
Multiplication Problems Using Fractions
    and Mixed Numbers   128
Finding the Unknown X in a Division
    Problem   130
Unknown X Problems Involving
    Division of Fractions   135
Section II Practice Problems   137
Answers for Practice Problems   138
Chapter 5 Problems   139

CHAPTER 6
MEASUREMENTS USED IN
VETERINARY MEDICINE   143

SECTION I METRIC UNITS   144

The Basics of the Metric System   144
Metric Units of Weight or Mass   146
Metric Units of Volume   148
Metric Units of Length   150
Combination of Metric Units to Describe
    Density or Concentrations   151
    Section I Practice Problems   152

SECTION II
COMMONLY USED HOUSEHOLD,
APOTHECARY, AND AVOIRDUPOIS
UNITS   153

Common Units   154
Conversions between Common
    Household Measurements   156
    Section II Practice Problems   157

SECTION III
CONVERTING BETWEEN
METRIC AND NONMETRIC
MEASUREMENTS   159

The Common Equivalents   159
Setting Up a Problem to Convert from
    One Unit to Another   160
Using the Proportion Method   161
The Cancel-Out Method   166
    Section III Practice Problems   170

Answers for Practice Problems   172
Chapter 6 Problems   174

CHAPTER 7
DRUG ORDERS AND
MEDICATION LABELS   179

SECTION I
THE DOSAGE REGIMEN   181

The Dose   181
The Route of Administration   183
The Dose Interval   184
The Dose Form   185
Handling Unclear Drug Orders   186
Section I Practice Problems   187

SECTION II
MEDICATION LABELS   188

The Drug Name   189
Dose Strength or Concentration   192
Dose Strength Listed as a Percent
    Solution   194
Dose Formulation and Number of
    Dose Form Units   196
Expiration Dates   199
Controlled Substances Labeling   199
USP and NF Label Designations   201
Hazard Warnings on the Label   203
Storage Information on the Label   204

Section II Practice Problems 205
Answers for Practice Problems 208
Chapter 7 Problems 211

CHAPTER 8
DOSE CALCULATION AND SYRINGE
MEASUREMENTS 219

SECTION I
THE BASIC DOSE CALCULATION 220

Converting the Animal's Weight for
Dose Calculation 220
Types of Doses Listed 222
Determining the Amount of Drug
for a Particular Animal 224
Determining How Many Units of
the Dose Form to Administer 225
When Tablet Doses Don't Come
Out Even 229
Dispensing Multiple Units of
Drug Form 230
The Most Common Calculation
Mistake in Dispensing
Multiple Units 233
Section I Practice Problems 237

SECTION II
DOSING WITH THE
HYPODERMIC SYRINGE 240

Types of Syringes Used in Veterinary
    Medicine   240
Syringe Units of Measurement   241
Measuring the Amount of Liquid in
    a Syringe   244
Section II Practice Problems   245
Answers for Practice Problems   251
Chapter 8 Problems   258

CHAPTER 9
CALCULATING INTRAVENOUS
INFUSIONS   269

SECTION I
INTRAVENOUS INFUSION OF
MEDICATION   270

Types of IV Administration Sets   270
Determining the Volume of Fluid
    Delivered   272
Converting Flow Rate between Time
    Units   279
Determining the Total Volume
    Delivered over Time   281
An Alternative Way to Determine
    Rate or Total Volume   284
Setting and Adjusting the IV Infusion
    Rate   287
Determining the Amount of Time
    for Drip Rate Observation   291
Section I Practice Problems   293

SECTION II
CALCULATING INFUSION
RATES WHEN ADDING DRUGS
TO IV FLUIDS   295

  Section II Practice Problems   299

SECTION III
CALCULATING STOP TIMES
FOR INFUSION RATES   301

The 24-Hour Clock   304
Converting Total Infusion Time   305
  Section III Practice Problems   309
  Answers for Practice Problems   310
  Chapter 9 Problems   314

CHAPTER 10
OTHER CALCULATIONS USED BY
VETERINARY PROFESSIONALS   323

SECTION I
RATIOS AND PROPORTIONS—
SOME ADDITIONAL POINTS   323

  Section I Practice Problems   326

SECTION II
CONVERTING TEMPERATURE
VALUES BETWEEN FAHRENHEIT
AND CELSIUS   327

  Section II Practice Problems   330

SECTION III
ROMAN NUMERAL
NOMENCLATURE   331

Writing Roman Numerals   332
Reading Roman Numerals   334
   Section III Practice Problems   336
   Answers for Practice Problems   337
   Chapter 10 Problems   340

MEDICAL MATHEMATICS AND DOSAGE CALCULATIONS

FOR VETERINARY PROFESSIONALS

CHAPTER 1

SELF-ASSESSMENT

Objectives

The student will be able to perform the following:

1. Conduct a self-assessment.
2. Identify areas needed for review.

In a medical situation, the most beneficial drug can be rendered worthless or dangerous if the veterinarian or veterinary technician does not accurately calculate the dose. As many veterinary professionals can testify, it is not enough to have a superficial understanding of dosage calculation, because superficial knowledge often fails in the crisis situation of an emergency. Therefore, it is important that the veterinary professionals have the basics of dose and dosage calculation firmly in their working memory.

Learning theory and common sense tell us that any mental activity practiced on a routine basis becomes second nature. It is important that the veterinary professional practice these routine dosage calculation procedures on a regular basis to ensure greatest accuracy whenever a dose needs to be administered.

Another obligation for any professional is to accurately define knowledge limits and to strengthen weaknesses in skills or knowledge. To help define areas of math and dosage calculation that need to be refreshed or reviewed, complete the following self-assessment exercises.

For each section in the self-assessment exercises that are identified as areas in need of review, work through the chapters and sections of this book referred to by that section of the self-assessment exercise.

SELF-ASSESSMENT EXERCISE

1. Add or subtract the following decimal numbers:

a) $1.5 + 2 =$

b) $1.9 + 9.7 =$

c) $4.55 + 7.43 =$

d) $0.52 + 0.09 =$

e) $0.003 + 1.0 =$

f) $5.5 - 2.5 =$

g) $6.0 - 3.9 =$

h) $13.125 - 1.50 =$

i) $0.251 - 0.095 =$

j) $0.00252 - 0.0009 =$

2. Multiple or divide the following decimal numbers:

a) $5 \times 2.5 =$

b) $3.0 \times 8.35 =$

c) $24.75 \times 12.35 =$

d) $0.02 \times 15.5 =$

e) $0.003 \times 0.0125 =$

f) $15 \div 2.5 =$

g) $2.5 \div 1.5 =$

h) $35 \div 0.5 =$

i) $0.25 \div 0.125 =$

j) $0.010 \div 0.0025 =$

3. Round the following decimal numbers to the nearest $\dfrac{1}{100}$ and nearest $\dfrac{1}{10}$:

a) $10.594 =$

b) 4.682 =

c) 1.233 =

d) 9.452 =

e) 23.675 =

4. Simplify the following fractions to their

lowest form (example: $\frac{6}{8} = \frac{3}{4}$):

a) $\frac{2}{10} =$

b) $\frac{4}{16} =$

c) $\frac{3}{12} =$

d) $1\frac{6}{8} =$

e) $5\frac{4}{32} =$

5. Add or subtract the following fractions:

a) $\frac{3}{4} + \frac{1}{4} =$

b) $\frac{1}{16} + \frac{3}{32} =$

c) $\dfrac{2}{5} + \dfrac{1}{6} =$

d) $1\dfrac{1}{2} + 2\dfrac{3}{4} =$

e) $4\dfrac{2}{3} + 5\dfrac{7}{8} =$

f) $\dfrac{1}{2} - \dfrac{1}{4} =$

g) $\dfrac{2}{3} - \dfrac{1}{6} =$

h) $1\dfrac{3}{4} - \dfrac{7}{8} =$

i) $3\dfrac{15}{16} - 2\dfrac{3}{8} =$

j) $45\dfrac{1}{5} - 33\dfrac{7}{8} =$

6. Multiply the following fractions:

a) $\dfrac{1}{2} \times \dfrac{1}{2} =$

b) $\dfrac{3}{4} \times \dfrac{1}{2} =$

c) $\dfrac{3}{4} \times \dfrac{12}{16} =$

d) $\dfrac{7}{8} \times 1\dfrac{1}{2} =$

e) $\dfrac{11}{16} \times \dfrac{3}{4} =$

f) $2\dfrac{3}{4} \times 4\dfrac{1}{2} =$

g) $5\dfrac{4}{7} \times 1\dfrac{3}{4} =$

h) $10\dfrac{3}{8} \times 9\dfrac{1}{3} =$

7. Divide the following fractions:

a) $\dfrac{1}{2} \div \dfrac{1}{4} =$

b) $2\dfrac{1}{2} \div \dfrac{1}{2} =$

c) $3\dfrac{3}{4} \div \dfrac{1}{16} =$

d) $22\dfrac{4}{8} \div \dfrac{2}{32} =$

e) $125 \dfrac{1}{5} \div \dfrac{4}{25} =$

8. Convert the following fractions to decimal numbers (example $\dfrac{1}{2} = 0.5$):

a) $\dfrac{2}{10} =$

b) $\dfrac{14}{28} =$

c) $\dfrac{3}{21} =$

d) $1 \dfrac{1}{2} =$

e) $4 \dfrac{5}{6} =$

f) $15 \dfrac{7}{16} =$

9. Convert the following decimal numbers to the common fraction (example $0.5 = \dfrac{1}{2}$):

a) $0.25 =$

b) $0.333 =$

c) 0.75 =

d) 0.125 =

e) 1.5 =

f) 2.500 =

10. Convert the following percentages to decimal numbers:

a) 25% =

b) 79% =

c) 100% =

d) 6% =

e) 0.2% =

f) 0.0087% =

11. Convert the following decimal numbers to percentages:

a) 0.5 =

b) 0.45 =

c) 1.00 =

d) 0.103 =

e) 0.90023 =

12. Convert the following percentages to commonly used fractions (example $50\% = \frac{1}{2}$):

  a) 25% =

  b) 75% =

  c) 33.3% =

  d) 10% =

  e) 80% =

13. Convert the following fractions to percentages (example $\frac{1}{2} = 50\%$):

  a) $\frac{3}{4} =$

  b) $\frac{8}{10} =$

  c) $\frac{15}{45} =$

  d) $\frac{10}{10} =$

e) $\dfrac{1}{1000} =$

14. What is 25% of 40?

15. A veterinarian wants to use 50% of 150 mg calculated dose. How much drug (in mg) would be given?

16. What percentage is 3 of 15?

17. A veterinary technician has drawn up 5 mg of the total dose of 20 mg of a drug to be given to an animal. What percentage of the total dose has been drawn up so far?

18. Solve for the missing X for each of the following:

a) $15 + X = 30 + 45$

b) $5 + 10 = 7 + X$

c) $X + 2.5 = 5.25 + 1.05$

d) $40 - X = 65 - 38$

e) $6.5 - 2.3 = 7.8 - X$

f) $X - 14.2 = 53.4 - 41.9$

19. Solve for the missing X for each of the following:

   a) $2 \times 6 = 3 \times X$

   b) $30 \times X = 120 \times 2$

   c) $X \times 25.5 = 43.2 \times 12.25$

   d) $25 \div 5 = 10 \div X$

   e) $300 \div X = 12.5 \div 8.125$

   f) $X \div 25 = 0.5 \div 0.75$

20. Solve for the missing X in the following proportions:

   a) $\dfrac{2}{8} = \dfrac{X}{16}$

   b) $\dfrac{4}{16} = \dfrac{3}{X}$

   c) $\dfrac{X}{32} = \dfrac{18}{9}$

   d) $\dfrac{12}{2} = \dfrac{X}{6}$

   e) $\dfrac{9}{X} = \dfrac{36}{12}$

SELF-ASSESSMENT EXERCISE ANSWERS

Check the following answers for each of the questions. Each answer section directs you to a section of this book that reviews how to perform each set of equations.

1. *FOR REVIEW OF THIS SECTION, SEE* Chapter 2, Sections I and II.

    a) 3.5

    b) 11.6

    c) 11.98

    d) 0.61

    e) 1.003

    f) 3

    g) 2.1

    h) 11.625

    i) 0.156

    j) 0.00162 or 1.62×10^{-3}

2. *FOR REVIEW OF THIS SECTION, SEE* Chapter 2, Sections III and IV.

a) 12.5

b) 25.05

c) 305.6625

d) 0.31

e) 0.0000375 or 3.75×10^{-5}

f) 6

g) 1.667

h) 70

i) 2

j) 4

3. FOR REVIEW OF THIS SECTION, SEE
Chapter 2, Section V.

a)	10.59	10.6
b)	4.68	4.7
c)	1.23	1.2
d)	9.45	9.5
e)	23.68	23.7

4. *FOR REVIEW OF THIS SECTION, SEE*
Chapter 3, Section I.

a) $\dfrac{1}{5}$

b) $\dfrac{1}{4}$

c) $\dfrac{1}{4}$

d) $1\dfrac{3}{4}$

e) $5\dfrac{1}{8}$

5. *FOR REVIEW OF THIS SECTION, SEE*
Chapter 3, Section II.

a) 1

b) $\dfrac{5}{32}$

c) $\dfrac{17}{30}$

d) $4\dfrac{1}{4}$

e) $10 \frac{13}{24}$

f) $\frac{1}{4}$

g) $\frac{3}{6} = \frac{1}{2}$

h) $\frac{7}{8}$

i) $1 \frac{9}{16}$

j) $11 \frac{13}{40}$

6. *FOR REVIEW OF THIS SECTION, SEE*
Chapter 3, Section III.

a) $\frac{1}{4}$

b) $\frac{3}{8}$

c) $\frac{9}{16}$

d) $1 \frac{5}{16}$

e) $\dfrac{33}{64}$

f) $12\dfrac{3}{8}$

g) $9\dfrac{3}{4}$

h) $96\dfrac{10}{12} = 96\dfrac{5}{6}$

7. FOR REVIEW OF THIS SECTION, SEE Chapter 3, Section IV.

a) 2

b) 5

c) 60

d) 360

e) $782\dfrac{1}{2}$

8. FOR REVIEW OF THIS SECTION, SEE Chapter 3, Section V.

a) 0.2

b) 0.5

c) 0.142857

d) 1.5

e) 4.833

f) 15.4375

9. *FOR REVIEW OF THIS SECTION, SEE*
Chapter 3, Section VI.

a) $\dfrac{1}{4}$

b) $\dfrac{1}{3}$

c) $\dfrac{3}{4}$

d) $\dfrac{1}{8}$

e) $1\dfrac{1}{2}$

f) $2\dfrac{1}{2}$

10. *FOR REVIEW OF THIS SECTION, SEE*
Chapter 4, Section I.

a) 0.25

b) 0.79

c) 1.00

d) 0.06

e) 0.002

f) 0.000087

11. *FOR REVIEW OF THIS SECTION, SEE*
Chapter 4, Section I.

a) 50%

b) 45%

c) 100%

d) 10.3%

e) 90.023%

12. *FOR REVIEW OF THIS SECTION, SEE*
Chapter 4, Section I.

a) $\dfrac{1}{4}$

b) $\dfrac{3}{4}$

c) $\dfrac{1}{3}$

d) $\dfrac{1}{10}$

e) $\dfrac{8}{10} = \dfrac{4}{5}$

13. *FOR REVIEW OF THIS SECTION, SEE*
Chapter 4, Section I.

   a) 75%

   b) 80%

   c) 33.3%

   d) 1%

   e) 0.1%

FOR REVIEW OF QUESTIONS **15** *THROUGH*
18, *SEE* Chapter 4, Section II.

   14. 10

   15. 75 mg

   16. 20%

   17. 25%

18. *FOR REVIEW OF THIS SECTION, SEE*
Chapter 5, Section I.

   a) $X = 60$

   b) $X = 8$

   c) $X = 3.8$

   d) $X = 13$

   e) $X = 3.6$

   f) $X = 25.7$

19. *FOR REVIEW OF THIS SECTION, SEE*
Chapter 5, Section II.

   a) $X = 4$

   b) $X = 8$

   c) $X = 20.75$

   d) $X = 2$

   e) $X = 195$

   f) $X = 16.67$

20. *FOR REVIEW OF THIS SECTION, SEE*
Chapter 5, Section II.

a) X = 4

b) X = 12

c) X = 64

d) X = 36

e) X = 3

DECIMAL NUMBERS

Objectives

The student will be able to perform the following:

1. Identify values of decimal places.
2. Add and subtract decimals.
3. Multiply and divide decimals.
4. Apply scientific notation.
5. Round numbers.

Drug dosages, concentrations of drugs in vials, and drug units are commonly expressed as decimal numbers. Therefore, it is imperative that the veterinary professional be able to accurately add, subtract, multiply, and divide using decimal numbers.

SECTION I
THE BASICS OF DECIMAL NUMBERS

RELATIVE VALUES

The decimal point, or "point," orients the reader to the values of the decimal number. Each space to the *left* of the decimal point increases by a power of 10. Therefore, the first space to the left of the decimal is "ones," the *next* space to the left is "tens," the next is "hundreds," and so forth.

Each space to the *right* of the decimal point decreases by a power of 10 *starting* with "tenths." The second space to the right of the decimal point is the "hundredths," the next is "thousandths," and so forth.

The number **7842.125** is shown below with each space's power of 10:

7	8	4	2	.
thousands	hundreds	tens	ones	decimal

1	2	5
tenths	hundredths	thousandths

Note that there are no "oneths" to the right of the decimal point.

READING DECIMAL NUMBERS ALOUD

When reading a decimal number aloud, there are two ways to communicate the number. Note these two ways for the number above:

"Seven-thousand, eight-hundred and forty-two and one-hundred and twenty-five thousandths"

"Seven eight four two point one two five"

The first method is more formal and represents the decimal point with the word *and*. All units to the right of the decimal place are read as units of the *farthest right* place. Therefore, in the number above, there were "125 thousandths." For the number "1.12," the value to the right of the decimal point would be read aloud as "12 hundredths" because the farthest right place that has a number in it is the hundredths place.

The second method for reading aloud or reporting decimal numbers conveys the information in a shorter, more concise manner. The numbers are read left to right, with the decimal point being spoken as *point*. No place values (hundreds, tenths, thousandths, etc.) are stated in this method. Therefore, "234.56" would simply be read aloud as "two three four point five six."

THE RULES FOR ZERO IN DECIMAL NUMBERS

If a decimal number is less than one, that is, there are only numbers in the places to the *right* of the decimal point, then the one's place contains a zero. For example, a number for twenty-five hundredths would be "0.25," and the number for one-hundred and twenty-three thousandths would be "0.123." The zero is not read aloud in the first method stated above, but it is read aloud in the second method. Therefore, the number "0.543" would be read aloud either way as follows:

"Five-hundred and forty-three thousandths"

"Zero point five four three"

Important Note: Adding the zero to the *left* of the decimal for numbers less than 1 helps prevent the decimal from being accidentally overlooked and a grossly excessive dose from being calculated! For example, if a dose is written as ".25 mg" and the decimal is accidentally overlooked by the veterinarian or veterinary technician administering the dose, then the animal is going to receive twenty-five milligrams, which is *100 times the intended dose!* Always add the zero to the left of the decimal for numbers less than 1 to emphasize the presence of the decimal point to someone reading your written instructions.

Generally, if a zero occurs at the farthest place to the right of the decimal, it is usually left off unless you wish to leave it simply to line up an equation or to mark the value of that farthest right place. For example, "1.50" or "1.500" would usually be truncated to "1.5." They represent exactly the same value (in both cases there are zero, or no, hundredths or thousandths).

Zeros between the digit in the farthest right place and the decimal point are *always* written in the decimal number. Therefore, "one and three hundredths" would be written as "1.03" and "forty-three thousandths" would be written as "0.043."

SCIENTIFIC NOTATION FOR DECIMAL NUMBERS

Notice that when you look at the numbers below quickly, it is not very easy to tell which number is different from the rest.

100000   100000   100000   1000000   100000

To reduce confusion in using very large or very small numbers, decimal numbers are often expressed in "scientific notation." Scientific notation expresses a numerical value as some number multiplied to the "power of 10." Below are several numbers expressed in scientific notation. Can you figure out the pattern for how scientific notation works?

$$10 \quad = \quad 1 \times 10^1$$

$$100 \quad = \quad 1 \times 10^2$$

$$20 \quad = \quad 2 \times 10^1$$

$$200 = 2 \times 10^2$$

$$250 = 2.5 \times 10^2$$

$$253 = 2.53 \times 10^2$$

The numerical value is expressed as a decimal number *times* 10 raised to a power (the superscripted number). 10 *raised* to the power of 1 = 10, 10 raised to the power of 2 is 100, and 10 raised to the power of 3 is 1000. Another way to think of it is that 10 raised to the power of 1 has one *zero* and 10 raised to the power of 3 has three *zeros*.

$$10^0 = 1$$
$$10^1 = 10$$
$$10^2 = 100$$
$$10^3 = 1000$$

Therefore, 3000 is actually 3×1000, and this can be expressed in scientific notation as 3×10^3. For the numerical value of 5,431, the scientific notation is expressed as 5.431×10^3.

To convert a scientific notation of 5.431×10^3 back to a decimal number, move the decimal point in 5.432 three places to the *right* because 10 is raised to the power of 3. Moving the decimal three places to the *right* gives us the original number of 5,431.

For numbers less than 1, the basic rules for writing scientific notation still apply;

however, we use the superscript of −1, −2, −3, and so forth to indicate the power of 10 used.

$$10^{-1} = 0.1$$
$$10^{-2} = 0.01$$
$$10^{-3} = 0.001$$
$$10^{-4} = 0.0001$$

The examples below illustrate how numbers less than 1 are expressed in scientific notation:

0.2	=	2×0.1	=	2×10^{-1}
0.25	=	2.5×0.1	=	2.5×10^{-1}
0.253	=	2.53×0.1	=	2.53×10^{-1}
0.03	=	3×0.01	=	3×10^{-2}
0.004	=	4×0.001	=	4×10^{-3}
0.0046	=	4.6×0.001	=	4.6×10^{-3}

To convert the form for a number expressed in scientific notation as "× 10 to a negative superscript" (e.g., 5×10^{-3}) into a decimal value, "move" the decimal to the *left* the same number of spaces as the superscript power. For example, to convert 5.75×10^{-4} back to its decimal form, we would move the decimal point 4 spaces to the *left*, placing zeros in any spaces needed.

$$5.75 \times 10^{-4} = 0.000575$$

←←←←

SECTION I
PRACTICE PROBLEMS
(Answers are at the end of the chapter.)

a) What digit is in the thousandths' location in the number 34623.8971?

b) Write the number: "twenty-five and sixty-nine hundredths."

c) Write the number: "thirty-three thousand, four hundred fifty-two and six hundred and forty-eight thousandths."

d) Write the number: "three six seven point two one zero four."

e) Write the number: "twenty-six thousandths."

f) Write the number: "zero point zero one two."

g) Write 3,673 in scientific notation.

h) Write 0.025 in scientific notation.

i) Write the decimal number for 5.39×10^5.

j) Write the decimal number for 8.32×10^{-2}.

SECTION II
ADDITION AND SUBTRACTION OF DECIMAL
NUMBERS

TIPS FOR ADDING AND SUBTRACTING
DECIMALS

When writing out decimal numbers for adding or subtracting by hand, errors can be eliminated by doing three things: (1) put the numbers in columns for adding, (2) line up the numbers with the decimal points in a vertical line, and (3) use zeros as "place-holders" to help you visually make sure the columns are aligned.

For example, adding 12.3 + 0.01 + 1.075 can be confusing if the decimals are not lined up vertically and would likely result in an incorrect answer:

$$12.3$$
$$0.01$$
$$+ \ 1.075$$

Lining up the decimals helps, but visually it looks a little odd:

$$12.3$$
$$0.01$$
$$+ \ 1.075$$

The use of zeros as placeholders to the right of the decimal number makes it easier for the eye to track down the columns correctly and add the appropriate numbers in each column:

$$
\begin{array}{r}
12.300 \\
0.010 \\
+\ 1.075 \\
\hline
13.385
\end{array}
$$

Remember that adding zeros to the far right side of the decimal number (as long as it is to the *right* of the decimal itself) doesn't change the value of the number.

Lining up the decimals in a column and adding zeros as placeholders are *very* important in subtracting decimal numbers by hand. For example, 12.35 – 1.255 *looks* odd with the decimals lined up vertically if no zero placeholders are used. It seems even odder when you try to subtract the "5 thousandths" from a blank space!

$$
\begin{array}{r}
12.35 \\
-\ 1.255 \\
\hline
\end{array}
$$

Putting the zero in as a placeholder makes the subtraction problem more familiar (borrow a "one" from the hundredths column and make the zero in the thousandths column a "ten").

$$\begin{array}{r} {}^{2\ 14\ 10} \\ 12.\cancel{350} \\ -\ 1.255 \\ \hline 11.095 \end{array}$$

SECTION II
PRACTICE PROBLEMS
*(Do by hand, and check with your calculator;
answers are at the end of the chapter.)*

a) 2.3 + 4.5 =

b) 13.56 + 4.32 =

c) 145.6 + 4.675 =

d) 0.23 + 1.034 =

e) 45.210 + 0.002476 =

f) 54.3 − 44.7 =

g) 362.65 − 4.29 =

h) 3.5 − 2.1567 =

i) 0.952 − 0.7 =

j) 12.133 − 0.09875 =

SECTION III
MULTIPLICATION OF DECIMAL NUMBERS

Unlike the necessity for lining up the columns of numbers discussed in addition and subtraction, multiplication of decimal numbers doesn't require vertical alignment. Instead, there are some simple rules for proper placement of the decimal in the multiplication answer (the "product").

The method is fairly simple. Multiply the two numbers together as if the decimals weren't there (that is, like a "regular" multiplication problem). Then count the *number* of digits (not their value) to the *right* of the decimal in all numbers that were multiplied in the problem. For example, if you were to multiply 2.3×4.55, there are a total of three digits to the *right* of the decimal point. When the answer (product) is calculated, the decimal is then placed, or moved, that number of spaces to the *left*. For our example of 2.3×4.55, the problem is solved as follows:

> There are a total of three digits to the *right* of the decimal in the two numbers being multiplied.

$$
\begin{array}{r}
4.55 \\
\times\,2.3 \\
\hline
1365 \\
910 \\
\hline
10.465
\end{array}
$$

←←← decimal point moved 3 spaces to the *left*

Note that by locating the decimal by this method, we don't need to line up the decimal point vertically in the multiplication problem.

The same rule stated above for writing decimal numbers in general applies to the decimal products of decimal multiplication. If the product is a number less than 1, you need to add a zero in the ones place to emphasize the existence of the decimal.

$$
\begin{array}{r}
90.2 \\
\times\, 0.01 \\
\hline
0.902
\end{array}
$$

←←← decimal point moved 3 spaces to the *left*

What happens if the *product* is only 3 digits long, but there are more than 3 digits to the right of the decimal in the problem? For example, 0.25×0.15 has four digits total to the right of the decimal point. But the raw answer, before placement of the decimal, comes out to 375, which only has 3 digits. In these situations, you need to add zeros to the *left* (not the right!) of the number until you have sufficient digits to place the decimal point. In the problem of 0.25×0.15, we need four digits to properly place the decimal in our product, so we place an additional zero to the *left* of our product 375 to give us 0375 as shown below:

$$
\begin{array}{r}
0.25 \\
\times\, 0.15 \\
\hline
125 \\
25 \\
\hline
0.0375
\end{array}
$$

←←←← decimal point moved 4 spaces to the *left*

Notice that the "emphasis" zero was put in the ones column in this case to call attention to the decimal point, even though a number with a zero in the tenths column would also call attention to the presence of the decimal point.

SECTION III
PRACTICE PROBLEMS
(Do by hand, and check with your calculator; answers are at the end of the chapter.)

a) $2 \times 4.5 =$

b) $1.3 \times 5 =$

c) $23.4 \times 4.15 =$

d) $35.167 \times 3.12 =$

e) $40.02 \times 18.15 =$

f) $5.002 \times 34.101 =$

g) $0.9 \times 8.2 =$

h) $0.123 \times 10.02 =$

i) $3.1002 \times 0.03 =$

j) $34.620 \times 0.023 =$

SECTION IV   DIVISION OF DECIMAL NUMBERS

Three terms are often used to describe division problems:

$$\text{divisor} \sqrt{\overline{\text{dividend}}} \; \overset{\text{quotient}}{}$$

dividend ÷ divisor = quotient

The dividend is the number being divided or split up by the divisor. The quotient is the answer to the division problem.

These are two forms of division problems that are set up in the same way.

$$5 \sqrt{\overline{10}} \; \overset{2}{}$$

$10 \div 5 = 2$

If you have a divisor (the number "dividing" the dividend) that is a decimal number and you are setting up the problem using the long-division bracket, move the divisor's decimal to the *right* until it becomes a whole number. Then move the dividend's decimal to the *right* the same number of spaces. For example, $82.5 \div 2.5$ put into the division bracket would look like this:

$$2.5 \sqrt{ 82.5 }$$

We then move the divisor's decimal point one place to the right to make it a whole number:

$$25. \sqrt{ 82.5 }$$
$$\rightarrow$$

moved one place to the right

Then move the dividend's decimal one place to the right also.

$$25. \sqrt{ 825. }$$
$$\rightarrow$$

moved one place to the right

Now divide the problem as you would any regular division problem, making sure you place the decimal in the quotient (answer) directly over the decimal in the dividend.

$$\overset{\downarrow}{25.\sqrt{\overset{\textstyle 33.}{825.}}}$$

If dividing $1.875 \div 0.15$, note how the decimal moves two places to the right to make the divisor a whole number:

$$0.15\sqrt{1.875}$$

$$015.\underset{\rightarrow\rightarrow}{\sqrt{\underset{\rightarrow\rightarrow}{187.5}}}$$

moved two places to the right

$$\overset{\downarrow}{15.\sqrt{\overset{\textstyle 12.5}{187.5}}}$$

Note: Sometimes the answer to a division problem terminates in a repeated number or series of numbers. For example, $100 \div 3 = 33.333333\ldots$ with the 3s continuing to infinity. Instead of rounding the number to 3.33334 (see "rounding" in the next section) we might elect to indicate the number, or pattern of numbers, that repeats by placing a horizontal line above the number(s). The examples below illustrate this use:

$$1.3333333... = 1.33\overline{3}$$

$$1.1272727... = 1.27\overline{27}$$

SECTION IV
PRACTICE PROBLEMS
(Do by hand, and check with your calculator; answers are at the end of the chapter.)

a) $5\sqrt{10.5}$ b) $8\sqrt{0.125}$

c) $0.3\sqrt{3.69}$ d) $1.02\sqrt{2.048}$

e) $0.8042\sqrt{3.01088}$ f) $33.0\sqrt{200.05}$

SECTION V   ROUNDING OF DECIMAL NUMBERS

Often in division and multiplication problems the answer appears as a very long decimal number. For example, $8 \div 1.23 = 6.504065$. If this answer were the number of milliliters (mL) to be injected into an animal, it would be impractical to attempt to determine where the mark for 6.504065 milliliters (mL) would be on the syringe. It then becomes necessary to round the number to the nearest tenth or hundredth, etc.

To round a decimal number, examine the digit to the *right* of the place to which you want to round your number. For example, if you want to round a number to the nearest tenths place, examine the digit in the hundredths. If you want to round a number to the nearest hundredths place, examine the digit in the thousandths place.

If the examined digit in the place is 5 or greater, round the number up one (i.e., increase the value of the number). If the examined digit is less than 5, the number remains the same. To illustrate this, we will round some decimal numbers to the nearest tenths.

Example: 3.87 rounded to the nearest tenth is 3.9

We examined the digit in the hundredths space (7) and found it to be greater than 5.

Therefore, the number in the tenths place was rounded "up" to the next digit (from 8 to 9).

Example: 3.84 rounded to the nearest tenth is 3.8

This time the number in the hundredths place was less than 5, so the number in the tenths column remained the same. Note that the number is *not decreased* when it is rounded "down."

Any digits that are to the right of the place to which you are rounding the number are truncated (dropped) when the number is rounded.

Example: 3.8923152 rounded to the nearest tenth is 3.9

Example: 3.8399999 rounded to the nearest tenth is 3.8

The same procedure is applied regardless of the place to which a number is being rounded. For example, we will round 6.53749 to the nearest whole number, the nearest tenth, the nearest hundredth, and the nearest thousandth. Check yourself to see if you agree with each rounding:

whole number 7 (digit in the tenths place is 5 or greater)

nearest tenth 6.5 (digit in the hundredths place is less than 5)

nearest hundredth 6.54 (digit in the thousandths place is 5 or greater)

nearest thousandth 6.537 (digit in the ten-thousandths place is less than 5)

SECTION V
PRACTICE PROBLEMS
(Do by hand, and check with your calculator.)

a) round $0.175 \div 2.3 =$ to the nearest hundredth

b) round $0.3 \times 6.732 =$ to the nearest hundredth

c) round 8.5002 to the nearest whole number

d) round 0.32897 to the nearest hundredth

e) round 0.0007023 to the nearest thousandth

f) round 1.03499 to the nearest hundredth

ANSWERS FOR PRACTICE PROBLEMS

SECTION I

a) 7

b) 25.69

c) 33,452.648

d) 367.2104

e) 0.026

f) 0.012

g) 3.673×10^3

h) 2.5×10^{-2}

i) 539,000

j) 0.0832

SECTION II

a) 6.8

b) 17.88

c) 150.275

d) 1.264

e) 45.212476

f) 9.6

g) 358.36

h) 1.3433

i) 0.252

j) 12.03425

SECTION III

a) 9

b) 6.5

c) 97.11

d) 109.72104

e) 726.363

f) 170.5732

g) 7.38

h) 1.23246

i) 0.093006

j) 0.79626

SECTION IV

a) 2.1

b) 0.015625

c) 12.3

d) 2.0078

e) 3.74394

f) $6.06\overline{21}$

SECTION V

a) 0.08   d) 0.33
b) 2.02   e) 0.001
c) 9   f) 1.03

CHAPTER 2 PROBLEMS

1. Write the numerical value (e.g., 35.09 pounds) described in each statement.

"I need twelve point three zero cubic centimeters (cc) given to this dog."
_____ cc

"Put twenty-five one hundredths of a gram into the IV solution."_____ grams

"We removed one hundred, thirty-two, and three tenths milliliters of fluid from his abdomen over the last 12 hours."
_____ milliliters

"The drug concentration was three thousandths of a mL."_____ mL

2. Calculate the total amounts (add or subtract) in each of the following statements.

"Add 12.4 cc and 3.5 cc to the IV fluids."
_____ cc

"Remove 0.5 mL from the 33.5 mL solution."_____ mL

"Combine the 4.5 grams, 3.2 grams, and 0.025 gram powders."

_____ grams

"Take out 3.5 tablets from the 55 you've dispensed."_____ tablets

3. Calculate the answers for the following decimal problems:

a) 10.35 + 0.03 + 2.005 + 13.025 =

b) 82.452 − 32.0031 =

c) 0.003 + 0.100 + 1.0214 + 0.0901 =

d) 0.03 − 0.00087 =

e) 19.0003 + 0.031001 + 2.83799 + 0.00679 =

4. Calculate the answers for the following decimal problems:

a) 3.12 × 0.01 =

b) 52.002 × 3.002 =

c) 96.01 × 38.909 =

d) 57.219 × 0.009 =

e) 86.030 × 1.029200 =

f) $166.003 \times 0.00399 =$

g) $0.0098 \times 3.92501 =$

h) $366.900 \times 3.009 =$

i) $352.88 \times 0.0097 =$

j) $0.010 \times 0.00392 =$

5. Calculate the answers for the following decimal problems:

a) $55.5 \div 5 =$

b) $7 \div 0.2 =$

c) $72 \div 1.002 =$

d) $19001 \div 32.021 =$

e) $0.002 \div 0.0003 =$

f) $15.0020 \div 2.0202 =$

g) $9.020999 \div 3.0299 =$

h) $0.0251 \div 0.0915 =$

i) $0.0528 \div 5.30005 =$

j) $5.30005 \div 0.0528 =$

6. Convert all of the answers in question 4 to scientific notation.

7. Convert all of the answers in question 5 to scientific notation.

8. Round the following numbers to the place indicated:

a) 32.092 nearest tenth

b) 1.17439 nearest hundredth

c) 4259.999 nearest thousand

d) 41.00195 nearest tenth

e) 819.273 nearest hundred

f) 9.93987 nearest hundredth

g) 0.009283 nearest ten-thousandth

h) 0.014263863 nearest millionth

i) 2.19283755 nearest hundred-thousandth

j) 5.555555 nearest thousandth

FRACTIONS

Objectives

The student will be able to perform the following:

1. Simplify fractions.
2. Add and subtract fractions.
3. Multiply and divide fractions.

Fractions are used in many medical situations. For example, a veterinarian may decide that he wants to "reduce the flow rate by half" or may decide to "divide the dose into thirds." The veterinary professional must be able to understand fractions, how they are calculated, and how to transition between fraction numbers and decimal numbers.

SECTION I FRACTION BASICS AND SIMPLIFYING FRACTIONS

NUMERATORS AND DENOMINATORS

A fraction is simply the way a whole of "something" is divided into small components. A "whole" tablet is split into two pieces, each piece is a fraction of the whole.

Our two smaller pieces would be represented by two fractions:

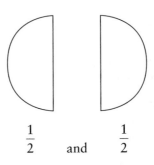

$$\frac{1}{2} \quad \text{and} \quad \frac{1}{2}$$

Figure 3.1 A whole split into halves

The top number is called the *numerator* and the bottom number is called the *denominator*. The denominator tells you into how many equal pieces the whole has been split. For example, when the tablet above was split into two pieces, the bottom number of the fraction (denominator) was a 2. The numerator tells you, "How many of the pieces do you have?" So if you split a tablet into two pieces and you take one of the two pieces, you have "1 of the 2 pieces" or "1/2" of the tablet.

If we divide a tablet as shown in Figure 3.2, we have four pieces. If you take one of the four pieces, you have "1 of the 4 pieces" or "1/4" of the tablet. If you take three of the four pieces, you have "3 of the 4 pieces" or "3/4" of the tablet.

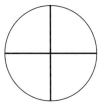

Figure 3.2 A whole split into four pieces

The larger the denominator, the smaller the piece (and the smaller the number value).

Notice that when we have our tablet divided into halves and another tablet of the same size divided into quarters, the fraction with the *larger* denominator (4) actually has pieces that are smaller in size than the fraction with the smaller denominator (2).

The numerical value for a fraction behaves the same way: 1/4 of a dose of medication is smaller than 1/2 of a dose of medication. Using the rule in the same way, 1/100 of a dose is much, much smaller than 1/10 of a dose. Other examples:

$$\frac{1}{3} \text{ is greater than } \frac{1}{4}$$

$$\frac{1}{5} \text{ is greater than } \frac{1}{10}$$

$$\frac{1}{16} \text{ is greater than } \frac{1}{32}$$

$\frac{2}{3}$ is greater than $\frac{2}{4}$

$\frac{3}{5}$ is greater than $\frac{3}{10}$

$\frac{10}{16}$ is greater than $\frac{10}{32}$

IMPROPER FRACTIONS, PROPER FRACTIONS, AND MIXED NUMBERS

If we had one whole tablet, and another half tablet, as shown below, we can see by adding up the "half tablets" that we would have a total of 3/2 tablets.

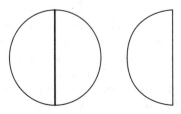

Figure 3.3 Mixed numbers

This amount (3/2) is called an *improper* fraction because the numerator (top number) is larger than the denominator. We usually don't write fractions as improper fractions (we would not say "give this animal 3/2 of a tablet"), instead we convert the improper fraction to a *mixed number*. A mixed number contains a whole number plus a *proper fraction* (numerator is *smaller* than the denominator).

To convert from an improper fraction to a mixed number, simply divide the numerator (top) by the denominator (bottom), use the number of even divisions as the whole number, and take the "leftover" as the remaining fraction. For example, the improper fraction 4/3 would be changed by dividing 4 by 3. We see that 3 goes into 4 only once, so our whole number in the mixed number answer is going to be 1. When 3 goes into 4, there is 1 left over, therefore the fraction of our mixed number is going to be 1/3. The final answer 1 and 1/3.

$$\frac{4}{3} = 1\frac{1}{3}$$

If the improper fraction were 5/3 , then the final answer would be 1 and 2/3 . Note that 6/3 results in an even division of 3 into 6, resulting in 2 with no leftover. Therefore, 6/3 = 2.

Sometimes it is necessary to convert from a mixed number back into an improper fraction. To do so, we simply reverse the process we just used. Instead of dividing, we multiply. To convert 1 2/3 back into an improper fraction, you multiply the denominator (bottom number) by the whole number, then add in the numerator (top number). For 1 and 2/3, we would multiply 3 (denominator) by 1 (whole number) to get 3, then add 2 (numerator) to get 5. The improper fraction answer would be 5/3.

FINDING EQUIVALENT FRACTIONS

Notice in our example of tablets divided into halves (1/2) and quarters (1/4) that if we took two of our quarter pieces and put them together, we would have reconstructed 1/2 of a tablet!

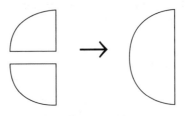

Figure 3.4 Finding equivalent fractions

This example illustrates what is meant by equivalent fractions. The two pieces of the quarter tablets together would be represented by the fraction 2/4 (two of the four pieces are together). We see visually that

$$\frac{1}{2} = \frac{2}{4}$$

The fractions 1/2 and 2/4 are said to be *equivalent fractions* because they numerically represent the same amount.

To create equivalent fractions, follow the rule:

"Whatever you do to the numerator, you must do to the denominator."

In other words, if you take the fraction 1/2 and multiply both the numerator and denominator by 2, you end up with the fraction 2/4.

$$\frac{1}{2} \times \frac{2}{2} = \frac{2}{4}$$

If you were to multiply the numerator and denominator of the 1/2 fraction by 3, 4, 10, or 2000, you would produce a whole series of fractions that were all *equivalent* to 1/2.

$$\frac{1}{2} = \frac{3}{6} = \frac{10}{20} = \frac{2000}{4000}$$

Therefore, in calculating equivalent fractions we are *not* changing the numerical *value* of the original fraction because we are multiplying the original fraction by 1. So, although equivalent fractions are different in *form* from the original fraction, they are not different in *value*.

SIMPLIFYING OR REDUCING FRACTIONS

If we have fractions like 2000/4000, they become rather difficult to work with. For example, how would you dispense 2000/4000 of a tablet? You certainly would not divide a tablet into 4000 pieces and then count out 2000 of them! Therefore, we need to simplify, or reduce, fractions by reversing the process we described above for producing equivalent fractions using the "Whatever you do to the numerator, you must do to the denominator" rule.

To simplify a fraction, determine if both the numerator and denominator can be *evenly divided* (no remainder left over) by the *same* number (called the *common divisor*). For example, if we have the fraction 2/4, we can easily see that both the top and the bottom of the fraction are evenly divisible by the number 2. So, to simplify the fraction, we divide the numerator by 2 and the divide the denominator by 2.

$$\frac{2 \div 2}{4 \div 2} = \frac{1}{2}$$

The fractions have equivalent values (two quarters of a tablet is the same as one half of a tablet), because we have divided the fraction by 2/2 or 1, and any number divided by one still has the same value. Again, the form is changed (2/4 to 1/2), but the value remains the same.

Fractions with large numbers may not immediately appear to be readily simplified, but if you check to see if both the numerator and the denominator are evenly divisible by the common prime numbers, 2, 3, and 5, you may find that the fraction can be simplified. Once you've simplified a fraction, check it again to see if it can be simplified further. In the example below, the student divided the numerator and denominator by 2 several times until the fraction was in its simplest form:

$$\frac{48 \div 2}{64 \div 2} = \frac{24}{32} \text{ then } \frac{24 \div 2}{32 \div 2} = \frac{12}{16} \text{ then}$$

$$\frac{12 \div 2}{16 \div 2} = \frac{6}{8} \text{ then } \frac{6 \div 2}{8 \div 2} = \frac{3}{4}$$

The common divisor for the numerator and denominator may change as you go through the steps of the reduction. For example, the fraction 18/24 can be partially simplified by dividing it by 2, but at the second step, it must be divided by 3 to reach its simplest form.

$$\frac{18 \div 2}{24 \div 2} = \frac{9}{12} \text{ then } \frac{9 \div 3}{12 \div 3} = \frac{3}{4}$$

Improper fractions are reduced by the same method. As an alternative, you can convert the improper fraction to a mixed number, and then reduce the fraction part of the mixed number while leaving the whole number untouched. For example, the improper fraction 6/4 is equal to the mixed number 1 and 2/4. Simplify the 2/4 to 1/2 and the final answer is 1 1/2 .

SECTION I
PRACTICE PROBLEMS
(Answers are at the end of the chapter.)

Write the equivalent fraction:

a) $\dfrac{1}{2} = \dfrac{?}{4} = \dfrac{?}{16} = \dfrac{?}{100}$

b) $\dfrac{1}{3} = \dfrac{3}{?} = \dfrac{5}{?} = \dfrac{12}{?}$

Reduce (simplify) the following fractions:

c) $\dfrac{4}{10}$ d) $\dfrac{6}{16}$ e) $\dfrac{24}{36}$ f) $\dfrac{36}{42}$

g) $\dfrac{72}{12}$ h) $\dfrac{73}{1}$ i) $2\dfrac{4}{8}$ j) $5\dfrac{24}{16}$

SECTION II ADDITION AND SUBTRACTION OF FRACTIONS

ADDING FRACTIONS

Adding fractions of tablets or medications is something veterinary professionals should be able to do accurately. It is not difficult to add two fractions that have common denominators (lower digit is the same in both fractions). Once the fractions have common denominators, the numerators (but *not* denominators) are added together:

$$\frac{1}{2} + \frac{1}{2} = \frac{2}{2} \quad \text{(which equals 1 whole)}$$

$$\frac{2}{5} + \frac{1}{5} = \frac{3}{5}$$

$$\frac{4}{10} + \frac{3}{10} = \frac{7}{10}$$

If, however, you have to add two fractions that do not have common denominators, it is not that simple:

$$\frac{1}{2} + \frac{1}{4} = ????$$

In this case, you need to convert the fractions to equivalent fractions (as discussed above) so that both fractions have the same common denominator. In the example above, you can easily see that we can convert 1/2 to the equivalent fraction 2/4 by multiplying both the numerator and denominator of 1/2 by 2 (using the rule: "Whatever you do to the numerator you must do to the denominator").

$$\frac{1}{2} \times \frac{2}{2} = \frac{2}{4}$$

The equivalent fraction 2/4 can now be added to 1/4 by adding the numerators (top numbers).

$$\frac{2}{4} + \frac{1}{4} = \frac{3}{4}$$

Note that a common beginner error is to add both numerators *and* both denominators! Remember to add (or subtract) only the top number (numerator) once the denominators are the same.

FINDING THE COMMON DENOMINATOR FOR MORE COMPLEX FRACTIONS

In more complex fractions it is not as obvious that there is a common denominator:

$$\frac{2}{5} + \frac{4}{7} = ????$$

In this case it appears that *both* fractions are going to have to be converted to equivalent fractions. To find the common denominator you could calculate a whole string of equivalent fractions for the first fraction, calculate another string of equivalent fractions for the second, and then see what common denominators there are between the two strings. However, a much easier way to find a common denominator between two fractions is to multiply each fraction by the denominator of the other fraction. For our example above, multiply both the numerator and denominator of the first fraction (2/5) by the denominator of the second fraction (7) to find its equivalent fraction. Then multiply the numerator and denominator of the second fraction (4/7) by the denominator of the first fraction (5) to find its equivalent fraction. This results in attaining, in one simple step, the common denominator for both fractions.

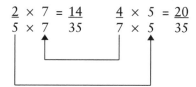

Figure 3.5 Finding the common denominator

The equivalent fractions can now be added because they have a common denominator.

$$\frac{14}{35} + \frac{20}{35} = \frac{34}{35}$$

Note that although the answer in our example can't be reduced, you should reduce the sum fraction if possible to a simpler form (for example, 20/25 reduces to 4/5).

SUBTRACTION OF FRACTIONS

Subtraction of fractions follows the same requirements as addition: you must have a common denominator for both fractions in order to carry out the mathematical operation. Finding the common denominator for both fractions is identical to the procedure described above.

For example, if you want to calculate 2/3 − 1/2, you need to find the common denominator for both fractions. Multiply each fraction (both top and bottom) by the denominator of the other fraction to find the common denominator:

$$\frac{2}{3} \times \frac{2}{2} = \frac{4}{6}$$

$$\frac{1}{2} \times \frac{3}{3} = \frac{3}{6}$$

Now the newly calculated equivalent fractions can be subtracted from each other by subtracting the numerators (top numbers).

$$\frac{4}{6} - \frac{3}{6} = \frac{1}{6}$$

ADDITION OF MIXED NUMBERS

Mixed numbers (whole numbers and fractions "mixed" together) can be added or subtracted by two methods. The *first method* involves converting the mixed number into an improper fraction, finding a common denominator for the fraction, then performing the addition or subtraction operation. For example, in calculating 1 1/2 + 3 3/4 , we first convert both mixed numbers to improper fractions (remember: an improper fraction has a numerator larger than the denominator).

$$1\frac{1}{2} = \frac{3}{2} \qquad 3\frac{3}{4} = \frac{15}{4}$$

$$\frac{3}{2} + \frac{15}{4}$$

We need to find the common denominator for the two components of the addition problem. In this case, we can easily see that multiplying the first fraction (3/2) by 2/2 converts the fraction into the equivalent fraction 6/4, which has the same denominator as the other component of the addition problem.

$$\frac{3}{2} \times \frac{2}{2} = \frac{6}{4}$$

Plug the equivalent fraction (6/4) into the equation and add the numerators to get the answer.

$$\frac{6}{4} + \frac{15}{4} = \frac{21}{4}$$

You can revert the improper fraction (21/4) back to the new mixed number by dividing 21 by 4 to get the new whole number and using the remainder of the division for the new numerator over 4.

$$\frac{21}{4} = 5\frac{1}{4}$$

In the *second method* you don't convert the mixed numbers to improper fractions at first. Instead, you focus on adding the "fraction parts" of the mixed numbers first, then add the whole numbers second. In our problem above we must still convert the 1/2 fraction in the 1 1/2 mixed number to a common denominator for the other fraction (3/4). To do so we multiply the top and bottom of the 1/2 fraction by 2.

$$\frac{1}{2} \times \frac{2}{2} = \frac{2}{4}$$

We now have the rewritten equation as:

$$1\frac{2}{4} + 3\frac{3}{4} =$$

Now add just the fractions in each mixed number together.

$$\frac{2}{4} + \frac{3}{4} = \frac{5}{4}$$

In this case we get an improper fraction. We convert the improper fraction to a mixed number (by dividing 5 by 4) to get 1 1/4.

$$\frac{5}{4} = 1\frac{1}{4}$$

Now that we have a sum for the fraction part of our mixed numbers, we add 1 1/4 to the whole numbers in our mixed number equation to find our grand total.

$$1 + 3 + 1\frac{1}{4} = 5\frac{1}{4}$$

Both methods are essentially the same. The major difference is when the improper fractions are reverted back to mixed numbers in the process. You should decide which of the two methods you are more comfortable with and consistently use that method.

SUBTRACTION OF MIXED NUMBERS

The first method described above for addition can be used for subtraction of mixed numbers.

Review of Method 1:

1. Convert the mixed numbers to improper fractions.
2. Find the common denominator for both improper fractions.
3. Subtract the fraction. (by subtraction of the numerators!)

The second method described in the section above, in which the mixed numbers are not converted to an improper fraction first, becomes a bit more complicated when you have to "borrow" a whole number in order to do the calculation. For example, in performing the following subtraction operation using the mixed numbers, we see that the fractions themselves can't be subtracted in their original form:

$$3\frac{1}{4} - 1\frac{3}{4} = ?$$

The 1/4 fraction is smaller than the 3/4 fraction, and therefore must be converted to another form before it can be subtracted. In this case we borrow a 1 from the whole number and add it to the fraction part of the mixed number.

$$3\frac{1}{4} \quad \text{becomes} \quad 2\frac{5}{4}$$

We added 4 fourths (4/4), or 1, to the fraction part of the mixed number to make it large enough to subtract the second fraction in our problem.

$$2\frac{5}{4} - 1\frac{3}{4} = ?$$

The value of the numbers involved has not changed, only the form. The problem is now solved by subtracting *the fractions* from one another to get the fraction component of the answer. The *whole numbers* are then subtracted from one another to get the whole number component.

$$2\frac{5}{4} - 1\frac{3}{4} = 1\frac{2}{4} = 1\frac{1}{2}$$

SECTION II

PRACTICE PROBLEMS

(Answers are at the end of the chapter.)

Solve the following problems:

a) $\dfrac{2}{8} + \dfrac{3}{8} =$

b) $\dfrac{3}{6} + \dfrac{6}{18} =$

c) $\dfrac{4}{48} + \dfrac{23}{24} =$

d) $\dfrac{3}{14} + \dfrac{35}{56} =$

e) $1\frac{3}{5} + \frac{49}{10} =$

f) $3\frac{14}{8} + 5\frac{25}{5} =$

g) $\frac{8}{16} - \frac{5}{16} =$

h) $\frac{4}{10} - \frac{7}{10} =$

i) $2\frac{3}{6} - 1\frac{4}{12} =$

j) $3\frac{12}{8} - 2\frac{4}{10} =$

k) $\frac{43}{12} - \frac{31}{18} =$

l) $\frac{38}{12} - 1\frac{14}{8} =$

SECTION III
MULTIPLICATION OF FRACTIONS

In some ways, the mechanics of multiplication and division of fractions is easier than fraction addition or subtraction. To multiply two fractions, simply multiply the numerators to get the product for the numerator of the answer, then multiply the denominators to get the denominator of the answer. For example, let's multiply 1/2 × 2/3.

$$\frac{1}{2} \times \frac{2}{3} = \frac{2}{6}$$

The numerators 1 and 2 were multiplied to produce 2 for the answer's numerator, and the denominators, 2 and 3, were multiplied to get the number 6 in the answer's denominator. Remember that it will often be necessary to simplify or reduce the answer to its simplest form:

$$\frac{2}{4} \times \frac{4}{6} = \frac{8}{24} \text{ which reduces to } \frac{4}{12} = \frac{2}{6} = \frac{1}{3}$$

MULTIPLICATION OF IMPROPER FRACTIONS

Improper fractions are multiplied together without having to change their form. As a general rule, if the answer is an improper fraction, you should convert it to a mixed number.

$$\frac{4}{2} \times \frac{8}{3} = \frac{32}{6} \text{ which is converted to}$$

$$5\frac{2}{6} = 5\frac{1}{3}$$

MULTIPLICATION OF WHOLE NUMBERS AND FRACTIONS

When multiplying a whole number by a fraction, you can convert the whole number to a fraction if you wish (e.g., 2 = 2/1, 5 = 5/1), or you can simply multiply the numerator of the fraction by the whole number. The equations below are equivalent in value.

$$3 \times \frac{2}{9} = \frac{6}{9} = \frac{2}{3}$$

$$\frac{3}{1} \times \frac{2}{9} = \frac{6}{9} = \frac{2}{3}$$

MULTIPLICATION OF MIXED NUMBERS

If you need to multiply one or more mixed numbers together, convert any mixed numbers to improper fractions, then multiply the improper fractions together. Don't forget to convert the improper fraction answer back to a mixed number and reduce the fraction if needed.

$$2\frac{1}{4} \times 3\frac{1}{2} = \frac{9}{4} \times \frac{7}{2} = \frac{63}{8} = 7\frac{7}{8}$$

A SHORTCUT FOR MULTIPLYING FRACTIONS

When multiplying fractions together, especially if multiplying several fractions together at once, the numerators and denominators can become very large, making the fractions difficult to work with. For example, multiplying $3/8 \times 4/7 \times 6/10$ gives the following answer:

$$\frac{3}{8} \times \frac{4}{7} \times \frac{6}{10} = \frac{72}{560}$$

The answer can be reduced to a smaller number, but it will probably take several reductions to get it down to its simplest form! The problem can be made easier by altering the form of the equation (but not its value). To do this we use a slight modification of our previous rule: "Whatever you do to the numerator, you have to do to the denominator." What we say now is that whatever you do to *one* of the *series* of numerators (in this problem, the 3, 4, or 6), you have to do to *one* of the *series* of denominators (the 8, 7, or 10).

Notice that in our series of numerators there is a 4 and in our series of denominators there is an 8. If we divided each of these numbers by 4 we would get a 1 and a 2 respectively ($4 \div 4 = 1$, $8 \div 4 = 2$). When we multiply the series of numerators together, we will replace the 4 with a 1, and when we multiply the series of denominators together, we will replace the 8 with a 2.

$$\frac{3}{\cancel{8}\,2} \times \frac{\cancel{4}\,1}{7} \times \frac{6}{10} = \frac{18}{140}$$

The answer is a lot simpler in form, but the equation could be made simpler still. For example, the 6 in the numerator series can be evenly divided by 2 and so can the 10 in the denominator series. Because we would be dividing both a numerator and a denominator in our series by the same number, this is a legitimate reduction. We replace the 6 with a 3 (6 ÷ 2 = 3) and the 10 with a 5 (10 ÷ 2 = 5). Then we multiply our series together.

$$\frac{3}{\cancel{8}\;2} \times \frac{\cancel{4}\;1}{7} \times \frac{\cancel{6}\;3}{\cancel{10}\;5} = \frac{9}{70}$$

The final answer is already reduced to its simplest form. Did we perform a legitimate mathematical calculation by doing this procedure? Let's check by reducing the original solution, 72/560, to its simplest form by dividing the numerator and denominator by 2 until we can't reduce it any further.

$$\frac{72}{560} = \frac{36}{280} = \frac{18}{140} = \frac{9}{70}$$

As you become comfortable doing fraction multiplication operations, try this shortcut as a way of simplifying your work.

In summary, to perform any fraction multiplication problem, make sure the numbers are in a fraction format, multiply the numerators, multiply the denominators, then convert to a mixed number and/or reduce the fraction as needed.

SECTION III
PRACTICE PROBLEMS
(Answers are at the end of the chapter.)

Solve the following problems:

a) $\dfrac{1}{4} \times \dfrac{1}{2} =$

b) $\dfrac{3}{8} \times \dfrac{5}{6} =$

c) $\dfrac{32}{3} \times \dfrac{3}{5} =$

d) $\dfrac{2}{5} \times \dfrac{16}{10} =$

e) $\dfrac{14}{4} \times \dfrac{26}{12} =$

f) $5 \times \dfrac{5}{6} =$

g) $\dfrac{32}{18} \times 4 =$

h) $2\dfrac{2}{3} \times 4\dfrac{5}{6} =$

i) $11\dfrac{7}{8} \times 23\dfrac{3}{5} =$

$$j) \quad \frac{3}{16} \times \frac{4}{9} \times \frac{12}{32} =$$

SECTION IV DIVISION OF FRACTIONS

THE RECIPROCAL

Before we actually talk about division of fractions, we need to introduce a new term that we will use in describing the division procedure. If we flip a fraction upside down, we create a *reciprocal*.

The reciprocal of 3/5 is 5/3. The reciprocal of 7/8 is 8/7.

Any fraction that is multiplied by its reciprocal equals 1.

$$\frac{3}{5} \times \frac{5}{3} = \frac{15}{15} = 1$$

Remember that whole numbers can be expressed as a fraction of that number over 1.

$$5 = \frac{5}{1}$$

Therefore, the reciprocal of a whole number is 1 over that whole number:

$$\text{Reciprocal of } 5 = \frac{1}{5}$$

DIVISION OF FRACTIONS

If we take a half of a tablet and divide it into two more pieces, we end up with 1/4 of a tablet.

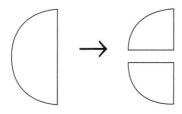

Figure 3.6 Division of fractions

What we did is to divide the 1/2 tablet by 2, which is represented by the equation:

$$\frac{1}{2} \div 2$$

In order to arrive at our answer of 1/4 of a tablet, what we actually did was multiply the first number (1/2) by the *reciprocal* of the second number. In this case the reciprocal of 2 is 1/2.

$$\frac{1}{2} \times \frac{1}{2} = \frac{1}{4}$$

Therefore, the key to dividing a fraction by a number is to convert the second number to its reciprocal and multiply the numbers together following the rules for multiplication from the previous section. So to find the answer for any fraction A/B divided by a whole number C, the following formula is used:

$$\frac{A}{B} \div C = \frac{A}{B} \times \frac{1}{C}$$

If we are dividing a whole number by a fraction, say 3 divided by 1/2, we would multiply the whole number by the reciprocal of the fraction. The reciprocal of 1/2 is 2/1.

$$3 \div \frac{1}{2} = 3 \times \frac{2}{1} = \frac{6}{1} = 6$$

To divide a fraction by a second fraction, we convert the second fraction to its reciprocal and multiply the fractions together. For example, to divide 2/3 by 1/2 we would actually multiply 2/3 by 2/1 to get our answer.

$$\frac{2}{3} \div \frac{1}{2} = \frac{2}{3} \times \frac{2}{1} = \frac{4}{3} = 1\frac{1}{3}$$

DIVISION OF MIXED NUMBERS

When dividing a mixed number by a fraction or dividing a number by a mixed number, always convert the mixed number to an improper fraction first. Once the mixed numbers are converted to improper fractions, multiply the first number by the reciprocal of the second fraction.

$$1\frac{1}{4} \div 2\frac{1}{2} = \frac{5}{4} \div \frac{5}{2} = \frac{5}{4} \times \frac{2}{5} = \frac{10}{20}$$

The final fraction is simplified or reduced and converted back to a mixed number if necessary.

SECTION IV
PRACTICE PROBLEMS
(Answers are at the end of the chapter.)

Solve the following problems:

a) $\dfrac{3}{4} \div \dfrac{1}{2} =$

b) $\dfrac{4}{5} \div \dfrac{1}{5} =$

c) $\dfrac{3}{8} \div 2 =$

d) $\dfrac{16}{32} \div \dfrac{2}{8} =$

e) $1\dfrac{1}{2} \div \dfrac{3}{8} =$

f) $\dfrac{1}{2} \div 4 =$

g) $3\dfrac{7}{8} \div 1\dfrac{3}{8} =$

h) $12 \dfrac{3}{16} \div 2 \dfrac{1}{8} =$

i) $125 \dfrac{3}{5} \div 5 \dfrac{1}{10} =$

j) $342 \dfrac{12}{16} \div 23 \dfrac{34}{64} =$

SECTION V
CONVERSION OF FRACTIONS TO DECIMALS

In order to calculate dosages using a calculator, we often convert fractions back into decimal numbers. Remember that decimal places to the right of the decimal point represent tenths, hundredths, thousandths, and so on. Therefore, if we have 2/10, the decimal equivalent would be 0.2. If you have 35/100, the decimal equivalent would be 0.35.

To find the decimal equivalent for fractions other than tenths, hundredths, and so forth, we first convert them to equivalent fractions of tenths, hundredths, thousandths, then make the transformation to the decimal number form.

$$\frac{1}{2} = \frac{5}{10} = 0.5$$

$$\frac{1}{5} = \frac{2}{10} = 0.2$$

There is another way to determine the decimal equivalent of a fraction without having to find its equivalent in tenths, hundredths, and so forth. By dividing the numerator (top number) by the denominator, you convert the fraction in one step to its decimal form.

$$\frac{1}{2} = 1 \div 2 = 0.5$$

$$\frac{4}{5} = 4 \div 5 = 0.8$$

$$\frac{8}{5} = 8 \div 5 = 1.6$$

For mixed numbers, convert the mixed number to an improper fraction first and then perform the same division to determine the decimal value.

$$1\frac{1}{4} = \frac{5}{4} = 5 \div 4 = 1.25$$

As you see in the problem above, you could also convert just the fraction, 1/4, to 0.25 and add it to the whole number, 1.

$$\frac{1}{4} = 1 \div 4 = 0.25$$

$$1 + 0.25 = 1.25$$

SECTION V
PRACTICE PROBLEMS
(Answers are at the end of the chapter.)

Convert the following fractions to decimal numbers:

a) $\dfrac{3}{4}$

b) $\dfrac{9}{10}$

c) $\dfrac{23}{35}$

d) $2\dfrac{7}{8}$

e) $\dfrac{48}{16}$

f) $23\dfrac{13}{32}$

SECTION VI
CONVERSION OF DECIMALS TO FRACTIONS

When you calculate a dose that must be translated into number of tablets or fractions of tablets, you must be able to convert from the decimal number you calculated to a fraction. For example, a student calculated a dose and found she had to give 0.75 of a tablet. How was she going to figure out how to cut the tablet up to give the appropriate dose?

To convert a decimal number to a fraction, start by writing it as a number over 10, 100, 1000 or whatever number corresponds to the "decimal place" the number occupies. For example, we know that 0.5 is 5/10 because the 5 is in the tenths place relative to the decimal. 0.75 is 75/100 because 75 occupies the hundredths place.

$$0.5 = \frac{5}{10} \qquad 0.75 = \frac{75}{100}$$

We then reduce the fraction to its simplest form by dividing the numerator and denominator by the same number (always try using 2, 3, 5, or other prime numbers).

$$0.5 = \frac{5}{10} = \frac{1}{2} \qquad 0.75 = \frac{75}{100} = \frac{3}{4}$$

If a decimal number is equal to or greater than 1, it can be converted to a mixed number (whole number and a fraction). First convert the number to the *right* of the decimal point to a fraction as described above, then use the number to the *left* of the decimal point as the whole number component of the mixed number. For example, convert 3.25 to a fraction:

$$0.25 = \frac{25}{100} = \frac{5}{20} = \frac{1}{4}$$

$$3.25 = 3\frac{1}{4}$$

ROUNDING FRACTIONS

In practical terms, you are going to have a hard time dividing a tablet of medication into 5/16 of a tablet. Therefore, in situations such as this, it is important to be able to round fractions to 1/2, 1/4, or 3/4.

When calculating a dose for a tablet, convert the decimal to the nearest 0.5 or whole number if you must round to the nearest half tablet, or convert the decimal to the nearest 0.25, 0.5, 0.75, or whole number if you must round to the nearest quarter tablet. You then convert the decimal to the fraction form as described above.

For example, after you have calculated a dose of drug for a dog, you find you need 4.30 tablets. The tablet is scored so that it can be easily divided into quarters. You know you are going to give 4 "whole" tablets, but you need to convert the 0.30 into the closest 1/4 tablet. Your next step is to determine which "quarter" 0.30 is closest to (0.25, 0.50, or 0.75). The 0.30 component of the decimal number is closest to 0.25; therefore we round 4.30 down (because we are decreasing the value of the number) to 4.25. You are going to use 4 1/4 tablets for this dose.

Suppose in the case above you had ended up with a dose calculation of 2.35 tablets, and the tablets were only readily divided in halves (not quarters). Because you have to round to the nearest half, the number has to be rounded to either 0.5 or to a whole number. In this case you see that 2.35 is closer to 2.50 (0.15 difference) than it is to 2.00 (0.35 difference). Therefore, you round 2.35 tablets "up" (because we are increasing the value of the number we are rounding) to 2.50. Because we know that 2.50 is the same value as 2.5, and that 0.5 = 1/2, we conclude that the appropriate dose is 2 1/2 tablets.

If you must round a fraction to the nearest 1/4 or 1/2, you first convert the fraction to a decimal number, round it to the nearest 0.25 or 0.5, then convert it back to the fraction. For example, if you are given the fraction 5/16 and need to round it to the nearest 1/4 tablet, you would divide 5 by 16 and get the decimal number 0.3125. You see that 0.3125 is closer to 0.25 (0.2500) than it is to 0.50 (verify this mathematically if you need to). We round 0.3125 down to 0.25, which is equal to 25/100, which then reduces to 1/4.

$$\frac{5}{16} = 0.3125 = 0.25 \ \text{(rounded)} \ = \frac{1}{4}$$

SECTION VI
PRACTICE PROBLEMS
(Answers are at the end of the chapter.)

Convert the following decimals to fractions and round to the nearest 1/4:

a) 0.25

b) 0.75

c) 0.225

d) 3.87

e) $23.67\overline{67}$

Round each fraction to the nearest 1/4:

f) $\dfrac{7}{16}$

g) $\dfrac{17}{64}$

h) $\dfrac{23}{5}$

i) $6\dfrac{2}{3}$

j) $23\dfrac{17}{32}$

ANSWERS FOR PRACTICE PROBLEMS

SECTION I

a) $\dfrac{1}{2} = \dfrac{2}{4} = \dfrac{8}{16} = \dfrac{50}{100}$ f) $\dfrac{6}{7}$

b) $\dfrac{1}{3} = \dfrac{3}{9} = \dfrac{5}{15} = \dfrac{12}{36}$ g) $\dfrac{6}{1} = 6$

c) $\dfrac{2}{5}$ h) 73

d) $\dfrac{3}{8}$ i) $2\dfrac{1}{2}$

e) $\dfrac{2}{3}$ j) $6\dfrac{1}{2}$

SECTION II

a) $\dfrac{5}{8}$ e) $\dfrac{65}{10} = \dfrac{13}{2} = 6\dfrac{1}{2}$

b) $\dfrac{15}{18} = \dfrac{5}{6}$ f) $4\dfrac{6}{8} + 10 = 14\dfrac{6}{8} = 14\dfrac{3}{4}$

c) $\dfrac{25}{24} = 1\dfrac{1}{24}$ g) $\dfrac{3}{16}$

d) $\dfrac{47}{56}$ h) $\dfrac{9}{40}$

i) $1\frac{1}{6}$

j) $1\frac{44}{40} = 2\frac{4}{40} = 2\frac{1}{10}$

k) $\frac{402}{216} = 1\frac{186}{216} = 1\frac{31}{36}$

l) $\frac{40}{96} = \frac{20}{48} = \frac{5}{12}$

SECTION III

a) $\frac{1}{8}$ f) $4\frac{1}{6}$

b) $\frac{5}{16}$ g) $7\frac{1}{9}$

c) $6\frac{2}{5}$ h) $12\frac{8}{9}$

d) $\frac{32}{50} = \frac{16}{25}$ i) $280\frac{1}{4}$

e) $7\frac{7}{12}$ j) $\frac{1}{32}$

SECTION IV

a) $1\frac{1}{2}$ b) 4

c) $\dfrac{3}{16}$

d) 2

e) 4

f) $\dfrac{1}{8}$

g) $\dfrac{31}{11} = 2\dfrac{9}{11}$

h) $\dfrac{195}{34} = 5\dfrac{25}{34}$

i) $24\dfrac{32}{51}$

j) $14\dfrac{142}{251}$

SECTION V

a) 0.75

b) 0.9

c) 0.657

d) 2.875

e) 3

f) 23.40625

SECTION VI

a) $\dfrac{1}{4}$

b) $\dfrac{3}{4}$

c) $\dfrac{1}{4}$

d) $3\dfrac{3}{4}$

e) $23\dfrac{3}{4}$

f) $\dfrac{1}{2}$

g) $\dfrac{1}{4}$

h) $4\dfrac{1}{2}$

i) $6\dfrac{3}{4}$ j) $23\dfrac{1}{2}$

CHAPTER 3 PROBLEMS

1. You have calculated the following amounts of medication to be given to different patients. Simplify each fraction.

a) $\dfrac{8}{100}$ d) $\dfrac{512}{768}$

b) $\dfrac{45}{125}$ e) $\dfrac{19}{57}$

c) $\dfrac{56}{128}$

2. Solve the following problems:

a) $\dfrac{4}{12} + \dfrac{7}{36} =$

b) $\dfrac{32}{16} + \dfrac{14}{28} =$

c) $\dfrac{13}{8} + 4 + \dfrac{8}{24} =$

d) $1\dfrac{1}{2} + 3\dfrac{3}{4} + 12\dfrac{7}{8} + \dfrac{24}{36} =$

e) $\dfrac{14}{28} - \dfrac{3}{14} =$

f) $8\dfrac{1}{4} - 5\dfrac{3}{4} =$

g) $12\dfrac{1}{2} - 9\dfrac{3}{4} =$

h) $\dfrac{32}{64} - \dfrac{45}{128} =$

i) $\dfrac{5}{10} \times \dfrac{18}{32} =$

j) $\dfrac{24}{36} \times \dfrac{18}{6} =$

k) $1\dfrac{1}{2} \times 3\dfrac{3}{4} =$

l) $12\dfrac{1}{4} \times 24\dfrac{1}{2} \times 4\dfrac{3}{4} =$

m) $\dfrac{1}{2} \div \dfrac{3}{4} =$

n) $3\dfrac{1}{4} \div 8 =$

o) $39\dfrac{12}{32} \div 5\dfrac{14}{16} =$

p) $\dfrac{125}{15} \div 7\dfrac{8}{50}$

3. Convert the following fractions to decimal numbers:

a) $\dfrac{7}{8}$ mL = _____ mL

b) $2\dfrac{3}{4}$ cc   = _____ cc

c) $\dfrac{39}{24}$ grams   = _____ grams

d) $45\dfrac{15}{18}$ mg   = _____ mg

4. Convert the following decimal numbers to the nearest 1/4 tablet:

a) 0.38 tablet   = _____ tablet

b) 1.799 tablets   = _____ tablets

c) 3.0921 tablets   = _____ tablets

d) 12.645 tablets = _____ tablets

e) 5.81022 tablets = _____ tablets

5. Over the next several days a dog is going to be on a decreasing dose of prednisolone tablets. The veterinarian has provided you with the daily doses below. Figure out how many tablets you need to dispense to cover the dosage regimen listed.

Days 1, 2, and 3	Give 1 1/2 tablet twice daily
Days 4, 5, and 6	Give 1 1/2 tablet once daily
Days 7, 8, and 9	Give 3/4 tablet once daily
Days 10–14	Give 1/4 tablet once daily

6. To determine how much drug you need to infuse into an animal intravenously, you follow the directions left by the veterinarian.

"The regular dose is 36 mg. Give 1/2 of the regular dose because of his bad kidneys. Add to that calculated dose 3 3/4 mg to compensate for the amount that sticks to the intravenous infusion set. But remove 1.825 mg from the total dose just to be safe."

How many mg of drug are you actually going to give intravenously?

PERCENTAGES

Objectives

The student will be able to perform the following:

1. Define percentages.

2. Convert percentages to decimal numbers and vice versa.

3. Convert percentages to fractions and vice versa.

4. Apply percentages to adjusting dosages.

Percentages are frequently used to describe how dosages are to be increased or decreased. It is important that the veterinary professional be able to understand percentages well enough to interpret drug orders, use percentages to properly calculate changes in drug dosages, and to accurately convert percentages to fractions or decimals.

SECTION I
DEFINITION AND USE OF PERCENTAGES

Percentage is another way of saying that we are looking at a certain number of items out of 100. In other words, if 5% of the tablets in a group of tablets are colored orange, we are saying 5 tablets out of 100 are orange in color. Therefore, percentage (%) is another way of saying "out of 100" or "for every 100."

CONVERSION OF PERCENTAGES TO FRACTIONS

Because percentages represent "X out of 100," we can represent any percentage as a fraction of "X/100." For example, 25% can be converted to an equivalent fraction form as follows:

$$25\% = \frac{25}{100} = \frac{5}{20} = \frac{1}{4}$$

Therefore, "25% of an administered dose of medication" would be equivalent to "1/4 of an administered dose of medication."

If the percentage has a value in tenths, hundredths, and so forth, then the decimal value in the numerator and the denominator are multiplied by a factor of 10 to make the numerator a whole number. An example is shown below:

$$12.5\% = \frac{12.5}{100} = \frac{125}{1000} = \frac{25}{200} = \frac{5}{40} = \frac{1}{8}$$

Therefore, 12.5% of an amount is equivalent to 1/8 of the amount.

CONVERSION OF PERCENTAGES TO DECIMALS

Percentages are best used in mathematical calculations when they are converted to an equivalent decimal number first. Because a percentage number is "X out of 100" (e.g., 25% = 25 out of 100), a percentage value is equivalent to "X hundredths" (e.g., 25% = 25 hundredths or 0.25). Therefore, to convert a percentage to its equivalent decimal value, simply *divide* the number by 100 or "move the decimal point two places to the *left*." The following percentages have been converted to decimals to illustrate this concept.

25%	=	0.25		
1%	=	0.01		
50%	=	0.50	=	0.5
100%	=	1.00	=	1
0.5%	=	0.005		

It is logical to assume that in order to convert a decimal number form of a percentage value back into a percentage, we *multiply* the decimal number by 100 or move the decimal point two places to the *right* and add a % sign.

0.15	=	15%
0.02	=	2%
1.00	=	100%
0.0045	=	0.45%

CONVERSION OF FRACTIONS TO PERCENTAGES

To convert fractions to their equivalent percentage forms, use the methods discussed in the previous chapters to first convert the fraction to its equivalent decimal number, then move the decimal point two places to the right. For example, the fraction 5/8 is converted to a percentage by the steps shown below:

$$\frac{5}{8} = 5 \div 8 = 0.625 = 62.5\%$$

Therefore, 5/8 of an amount is equivalent to 62.5% of the amount.

SECTION I
PRACTICE PROBLEMS
(Answers are at the end of the chapter.)

1) Convert the following percentages to decimals:

a) 50%

b) 25%

c) 1.5%

d) 0.7%

e) 10.23%

f) 0.085%

g) 125%

h) 203.55%

2) Convert the decimals to percentages:

a) 0.75   e) 0.10

b) 0.125   f) 0.08125

c) 0.015   g) 1.25

d) 0.0035   h) 3.001

3) Convert the following percentages to fractions:

a) 50%   e) 0.10%

b) 25%   f) 0.025%

c) 12.5%   g) 125.00%

d) 1.0%   h) 15.25%

4) Convert the following fractions to percentages:

a) 1/2   e) 1/10

b) 3/4   f) 2/5

c) 1/8   g) 9/32

d) 1/32   h) 24/56

SECTION II
USING PERCENTAGES TO SOLVE PROBLEMS

Veterinary professionals need to be careful in how they use the word *percentage* in verbal or written orders. Here are some examples of ways the word *percentage* might be phrased in adjusting a dose:

1) How many mg is 20% of a 100 mg dose?

2) How much drug will I give if I want to use 75% of the original 100 mg dose?

3) How many mg are we giving if we use 120% of the 100 mg dose?

4) What amount of a 100 mg dose do we use if we increase or decrease it by 20%?

5) How much of the 200 mg is left if 20% is removed?

6) What percentage of 100 mg is 20 mg?

7) What percentage is 20 mg of 100 mg?

Each of these sentences asks something slightly different. It is important that the veterinary professional be able to convert written or verbal orders conveyed in this way into the correct mathematical equations to ensure proper calculations or dosage adjustment.

FINDING THE PERCENTAGE OF A WHOLE

In the first sentence, "How many mg is 20% of a 100 mg dose?" we are attempting to find out the number of milligrams found in the fraction (20%) of the whole (100 mg). Remember that the percentage in this problem represents a certain fraction of the whole; therefore, if we multiply the whole (100 mg) by the "fraction" (20%), we should be able to find out the "worth" or amount of the fractional amount. To do this, first convert the percentage to its equivalent decimal number then multiply the whole by this decimal number.

$$20\% = 0.20 = 0.2$$
(decimal equivalent of 20%)

$$0.2 \times 100 \text{ mg} = 20 \text{ mg}$$

Remember how our original definition of percentage was the number of items "out of 100 items"? We see in the problem above that 20% indeed equals 20 mg out of 100 mg.

Therefore, to find the amount represented by the percentage value (the fractional amount of the whole) we can use the following general equation:

Percentage × Whole Amount = Fractional Amount

In the second sentence of our examples, "How much drug will I give if I want to use 75% of the original 100 mg dose?" we are attempting to identify the quantity of the fractional amount represented by the 75%. Therefore, we can apply the same method that we used above:

75% = 0.75

0.75 × 100 mg = 75 mg

The third sentence, "How many mg are we giving if we use 120% of the 100 mg dose?" seems to contradict the definition of percentages because we are talking about "120 out of 100"! This terminology is often used to indicate the need to find a number greater than the original whole. Another mathematically correct way of putting it would be to say that we're looking for an amount that is 100% of the original plus 20% of the original (100% + 20% = 120%). Instead of doing a multistep calculation, we can convert the 120% into a decimal using the same rules for conversion that we've used before, then multiply the original whole by the decimal.

120% = 1.20 = 1.2
(remember that 100% = 1 whole)

1.2 × 100 mg = 120 mg

Here are several examples of similar statements and the mathematical calculations that would be used to determine the answer to the question.

How many mg is 50% of a 200 mg dose?

0.5×200 mg = 100 mg

If we use 25% of the original 600 mg dose, how much will be used?

0.25×600 mg = 150 mg

How much drug will I give if I want to use 45% of the original 300 mg dose?

0.45×300 mg = 135 mg

If I have 200 mg and want to give 75% of the dose, what dose am I giving?

0.75×200 mg = 150 mg

How many mg are we giving if we use 200% of the 50 mg dose?

$2.00 = 2$

2×50 mg = 100 mg

SUBTRACTING OR ADDING THE PERCENTAGE OF THE WHOLE

The fourth sentence in our list of example statements asks a slightly different question: "What amount of a 100 mg dose do we use if we increase or decrease it by 20%?"

This question really has two components to it. First, we have to determine the amount of the percentage, then we have to adjust the dose by that amount. To perform this calculation, we begin with the same procedure of converting the percentage into a decimal then calculating the percentage amount:

0.20×100 mg = 20 mg

If we are increasing the dose by 20%, we then add this amount to the whole amount to get the new dose.

20 mg + 100 mg = 120 mg

The same principles apply to decreasing the dose by 20%, except that you subtract the calculated amount from the whole.

100 mg − 20 mg = 80 mg

The sentence in the example statements, "How much of the 200 mg is left if 20% is removed?" is asking how much of the whole will be left over after 20% is removed. Once again, we calculate the amount and subtract it from the whole.

$$20\% = 0.2$$

$$0.2 \times 200 \text{ mg} = 40 \text{ mg}$$

$$200 \text{ mg} - 40 \text{ mg} = 160 \text{ mg}$$

DETERMINING PERCENTAGES REPRESENTED BY THE FRACTIONAL COMPONENT

In two sentences in the examples, the student is asked to determine what percentage of the whole is represented by the fractional amount:

What percentage of 100 mg is 20 mg?

What percentage is 20 mg of 100 mg?

A direct way to answer these questions is to set up a fraction, convert it to a decimal number, and then convert to a percentage.

$$\text{Fraction} = \frac{20 \text{ mg}}{100 \text{ mg}}$$

Convert to a decimal by dividing the numerator by the denominator.

20 mg ÷ 100 mg = 0.2

Convert to a percentage (move decimal point two places to the right.)

0.2 = 0.20 = 20%

Therefore 20 mg is 20% of 100 mg.

The same procedure is used for the following:

What percentage of 400 mg is 50 mg?

$$\frac{50 \text{ mg}}{400 \text{ mg}}$$

50 ÷ 400 = 0.125

0.125 = 12.5%

What percentage is 25 mg of 200 mg?

$$\frac{25 \text{ mg}}{200 \text{ mg}}$$

25 ÷ 200 = 0.125

0.125 = 12.5%

By practicing working with percentages on a regular basis, you should get to the point where setting up these equations to accurately solve dosing problems is almost second nature.

SECTION II
PRACTICE PROBLEMS
(Answers are at the end of the chapter.)

1) How many mg is 12% of a 50 mg dose?

2) How much drug will I give if I want to use 30% of the original 60 mg dose?

3) How many mg are we giving if we use 150% of the 75 mg dose?

4) What amount of a 250 mg dose do we add if we increase it by 20%?

5) What dose do we use if we decrease a 200 mg dose by 10%?

6) How much of the 25 mg is left if 5% is removed?

7) What percentage of 500 mg is 5 mg?

8) What percentage is 12.5 mg of 37.5 mg?

9) A dog on digoxin (heart medication) has shown signs of drug toxicity. Therefore the veterinarian wants to decrease the 0.125 mg dose by 20%. What is the new dose?

10) A dog with epilepsy (seizures) is not well controlled at a dose of 60 mg every 12 hours. The veterinarian decides that the dose should be given at 175% of the cur-

rent dose. How much drug will this dog receive every 12 hours?

ANSWERS FOR PRACTICE PROBLEMS

SECTION I

1.
a) 0.50   b) 0.25   c) 0.015   d) 0.007

e) 0.1023   f) 0.00085   g) 1.25   h) 2.0355

2.
a) 75%   b) 12.5%   c) 1.5%   d) 0.35%

e) 10%   f) 8.125%   g) 125%   h) 300.1%

3.
a) 1/2   b) 1/4   c) 1/8   d) 1/100

e) 1/1000 f) 1/4000   g) 11/4   h) 61/400

4.
a) 50%   b) 75%   c) 12.5%   d) 3.125%

e) 10%   f) 40%   g) 28.125% h) 42.86%

SECTION II

1. 6 mg   6. 23.75 mg

2. 18 mg   7. 1%

3. 112.5 mg   8. 33.3%

4.   50 mg   9.   0.1 mg

5.   180 mg   10.   105 mg

CHAPTER 4 PROBLEMS

1) If you are going to increase a dose by 25%, you will need to multiply the dose by what decimal number?

2) The number of tablets to be dispensed to Mr. Jones was decreased by the following equation: 45 tablets ¥ 0.33 = 15 tablets. What percentage is 15 of 45?

3) If you have to decrease the amount of intravenous fluid by 1/4, by what percentage is the amount of fluid being decreased?

4) If you are told to decrease an intravenous dose of drug to 1/10 of the original 250 mg dose, how much drug will you give?

5) How many mg is 15% of a 200 mg dose of amoxicillin? If we decreased the dose by 15%, what would the new dose of amoxicillin be?

6) In liver disease, the dose of some drugs metabolized by the liver needs to be reduced by 25%. If one of these drugs is normally dosed at 120 mg, what will be the new adjusted dose if the animal has liver disease?

7) The drug was decreased from 250 mg to 125 mg. What percentage was the dose decreased? What fraction represents this decrease? What would you multiply 250 by to get 125?

8) An animal was on 25 mg of prednisone a day last week and then was bumped up to 75 mg a day. What percentage increase of dose is this? What fraction represents this increase? What would you multiply 25 by to get 75?

9) You started out giving 2000 mL of fluid. Four hours later 250 mL is left. By what percentage has the original amount been reduced? What percentage of the fluid is left?

10) There is only 10% of the original 30 mL vial left. How many mL are left? How much has been removed?

11) The dose of the beta-blocker drug (antiarrhythmia heart drug) is now 200% of what it was 3 days ago. If the original dose was X mg, how would you calculate the current dose based upon the old dose of "X" amount?

12) Because of the decreased renal function, the 600 mg dose of gentamicin needs to be decreased by 12.5%. How much gentamicin will this animal be receiving?

CHAPTER 5

SOLVING FOR THE UNKNOWN VALUE X

Objectives

The student will be able to perform the following:

1. Set up an equation to find an Unknown value X when given two or three values and their relationship to X.
2. Perform the mathematical calculations necessary to identify the value of X.
3. Apply methods for solving X to dosage calculations.

In most dosage calculations, you will be given certain information plus a description of the relationship between the given information and other variables. You will then be required to set up a calculation so that you determine a missing value. For example, the given information may be the animal's weight (e.g., 15 kg), the relationship between variables would be a drug dose (e.g., 10 mg per kg of body weight), and the missing value would be the dose to be administered to an animal of this weight. It is very important to have a solid grasp of how to accurately set up these equations and perform the mathematical operations

111

necessary to determine the missing value of Unknown value "X."

SECTION I
FINDING THE VALUE OF THE UNKNOWN X IN ADDITION AND SUBTRACTION

The basic steps in finding the Unknown X in addition and subtraction problems can be extended to do multiplication and division Unknown problems as well as dosage calculations. Therefore, understanding the fundamentals of how to solve for addition and subtraction Unknowns will greatly aid the student in understanding more complex problems.

ANALYZING THE PROBLEM AND SETTING UP THE EQUATION

Let's say we were compounding two powdered forms of Drug A and Drug B together in a single capsule. We were able to add 25 mg of Drug A and 40 mg of Drug B in the first capsule. Then let's say the amount of Drug A was to be increased by twice the original amount A (double 25 mg to 50 mg). How much of Drug B would now fit in that same capsule with the increased amount of Drug A?

In analyzing this type of problem we always place the *known* values from one set of conditions on one side of the equal sign, and then place any remaining known value(s) and the Unknown X from the other set of conditions on the other side. In the example above, we know that the first condition of known values is the total amount of Drugs A and B in the first capsule formulation. The second set of conditions is the amount of Drugs A and B placed into the second capsule formulation. Because the values in both conditions must equal each other, we set up the equation to look like this:

Amount of Drug A1 + Amount of Drug B1 = Amount of Drug A2 + Amount of Drug B2

We now can plug the given known values into the equation and identify what value is missing, which will be designated our Unknown value X.

25 mg (Drug A1) + 40 mg (Drug B1) = 50 mg (Drug A2) + X mg (Drug B2)

Once the equation of conditions has been set up, the next step is to isolate the Unknown on one side of the equal sign. By doing this we will be left with a series of mathematical operations on one side of the equal sign, which, when performed, will give us the value for our Unknown.

In order to isolate the Unknown to one

side of the equation, we have to move all the known values (such as the 50 mg in the example) to the other side of the equation. How do we do this?

MOVING THE VALUES FROM ONE SIDE OF THE EQUATION TO THE OTHER

The equal sign acts like the fulcrum or balance point on a scale. Therefore, anything that is done to one side of the equation must be done to the other to maintain the equality (the "balance") between the two sides. If we take away a value of 15 from one side of an equation, we have to take away a value of 15 from the other to maintain the mathematical "balance" of the equation.

We can use this fact to move any known values from the side of the equation with the Unknown value to the other side of the equal sign, leaving the Unknown by itself on one side of the equation. In our example we see that we need to move the 50 mg value to the other side of the equation in order to leave the Unknown alone on the right (mg of Drug B in capsule 2).

25 mg + 40 mg = 50 mg + X mg (Drug B2)

Notice we can make the 50 mg "disappear" by subtracting 50 mg from itself.

25 mg + 40 mg = 50 mg – 50 mg + X mg (Drug B2)

25 mg + 40 mg = 0 + X mg (Drug B2)

25 mg + 40 mg = X mg (Drug B2)

But remember that whatever we do to one side of the equation we must do to the other. Therefore if we subtracted 50 mg from one side, then we must subtract 50 mg from the other side of the equation.

25 mg + 40 mg – 50 mg = X mg (Drug B2)

We now have a mathematical equation for solving the missing Unknown value X.

65 mg – 50 mg = X mg

15 mg = X mg

Therefore, the amount of Drug B placed in the second capsule was 15 mg. To check this answer to see if it is correct, replace the Unknown X in the original equation with 15 mg and see if this results in the same value on either side of the equation.

25 mg + 40 mg = 50 mg + X mg

25 mg + 40 mg = 50 mg + 15 mg

$$65 \text{ mg} = 65 \text{ mg}$$

Because both sides of the equation are equal, our answer must have been correct.

To review the steps for determining an Unknown value X in an addition equation:

1. Set up an equation with the two sets of conditions on either side of the equal sign.

2. Move any known values from the side with the Unknown X to the other side of the equation by converting the known values to zero and making sure the same amounts are subtracted from both sides of the equation.

3. Perform the mathematical operation on the rearranged equation.

Note how these two examples are set up and performed to identify the Unknown value of X.

Example:

$$45 \text{ mL} + X \text{ mL} = 35 \text{ mL} + 50 \text{ mL}$$

$$45 \text{ mL} - 45 \text{ mL} + X \text{ mL} = 35 \text{ mL} + 50 \text{ mL} - 45 \text{ mL}$$

$$0 \text{ mL} + X \text{ mL} = 35 \text{ mL} + 50 \text{ mL} - 45 \text{ mL}$$

$$X \text{ mL} = 85 \text{ mL} - 45 \text{ mL}$$

$$X \text{ mL} = 40 \text{ mL}$$

Check it:

$$45 \text{ mL} + 40 \text{ mL} = 35 \text{ mL} + 50 \text{ mL}$$

$$85 \text{ mL} = 85 \text{ mL}$$

Example:

23 kg + 37.4 kg + 28.75 kg = 63.4 kg + 12.4 kg + X kg

23 kg + 37.4 kg + 28.75 kg – 63.4 kg – 12.4 kg = 63.4 kg – 63.4 kg + 12.4 kg – 12.4 kg + X kg

23 kg + 37.4 kg + 28.75 kg – 63.4 kg – 12.4 kg = 0 kg + 0 kg + X kg

23 kg + 37.4 kg + 28.75 kg – 63.4 kg – 12.4 kg = X kg

13.35 kg = X kg

Check it:

23 kg + 37.4 kg + 28.75 kg = 63.4 kg + 12.4 kg + 13.35 kg

$$89.15 \text{ kg} = 89.15 \text{ kg}$$

MOVING NEGATIVE NUMBERS OF
UNKNOWN X IN SUBTRACTION

In the example shown below, we have a subtraction problem. In effect, we have a negative 30 kilograms (– 30 kg) and a negative Unknown X (– X) in the equation.

$$45 \text{ kg} - 30 \text{ kg} = 60 \text{ kg} - X$$

We still need to isolate the Unknown X by itself on one side of the equation, but observe what happens if we use the same technique as described above to isolate the Unknown X by moving the 60 kg to the other side of the equation.

$$45 \text{ kg} - 30 \text{ kg} - 60 \text{ k} = 60 \text{ kg} - 60 \text{ kg} - X$$

$$- 45 = - X$$

We end up with a negative 45 equal to a negative X. Although we could multiply both sides by –1 to change the X value to a positive X, it would be easier if we didn't have to deal with a –X value in the first place.

The way to avoid this problem is to first rearrange the equation so that the Unknown X is a positive value.

To do this, instead of moving the 60 kg to the other side of the equation to isolate the Unknown X, move the –X to the opposite side of the equation instead. To make the –X "disappear" from one side of the equation and reappear on the other side, we *add* X to either side of the equation.

$$45 \text{ kg} - 30 \text{ kg} = 60 \text{ kg} - X$$

$$45 \text{ kg} - 30 \text{ kg} + X = 60 \text{ kg} - X + X$$

$$45 \text{ kg} - 30 \text{ kg} + X = 60 \text{ kg} - 0$$

$$45 \text{ kg} - 30 \text{ kg} + X = 60 \text{ kg}$$

Now we need to isolate the Unknown X on one side of the equation. To do this, we need to move the 45 kg and the negative 30 kg (– 30 kg) to the opposite side. By adding a negative 45 and a *positive* 30 kg to each side, we should end up with just the Unknown X on the left side of the equation.

$$45 \text{ kg} - 30 \text{ kg} + X = 60 \text{ kg}$$

$$45 \text{ kg} - 45 \text{ kg} + 30 \text{ kg} - 30 \text{ kg} + X = 60 \text{ kg} - 45 \text{ kg} + 30 \text{ kg}$$

$$0 \text{ kg} + 0 \text{ kg} + X = 15 \text{ kg} + 30 \text{ kg}$$

$$X = 45 \text{ kg}$$

Check it!

$$45 \text{ kg} - 30 \text{ kg} = 60 \text{ k} - 45 \text{ kg}$$

$$15 \text{ kg} = 15 \text{ kg}$$

The three essential steps to set up and solve these Unknown problems are

1. Rearrange the equation, if necessary, to make the Unknown X a *positive* value.

2. Isolate the positive Unknown X on one side of the equation.

3. Perform the mathematical operation on the rearranged equation.

By remembering these three steps, we can solve problems in which the equation involves a mixture of positive and negative values. The problem below may appear complicated at first, but by following the two essential steps, the problem can be set up to be easily solved.

$$- X \text{ mL} + 25 \text{ mL} - 10 \text{ mL} = - 20 \text{ mL}$$

The Unknown X value is negative, so we need to move it to the other side of the equation to make it positive.

$$X \text{ mL} - X \text{ mL} + 25 \text{ mL} - 10 \text{ mL} = X \text{ mL} - 20 \text{ mL}$$

$$0 + 25 \text{ mL} - 10 \text{ mL} = X \text{ mL} - 20 \text{ mL}$$

$$25 \text{ mL} - 10 \text{ mL} = X \text{ mL} - 20 \text{ mL}$$

Now isolate the positive Unknown value X.

$$25 \text{ mL} - 10 \text{ mL} + 20 \text{ mL} = X \text{ mL} - 20 \text{ mL} + 20 \text{ mL}$$

25 mL – 10 mL + 20 mL = X mL – 0

25 mL – 10 mL + 20 mL = X mL

15 mL + 20 mL = X mL

35 mL = X mL

Check it!

– X mL + 25 mL – 10 mL = – 20 mL

– 35 mL + 25 mL – 10 mL = – 20 mL

– 10 mL – 10 mL = – 20 mL

– 20 mL = – 20 mL

The values are the same on either side of the equation; therefore, the answer must be correct. By remembering and applying the three essential steps in solving for the Unknown X, even relatively complex equations can be solved.

SECTION I
PRACTICE PROBLEMS
(Answers are at the end of the chapter.)

Solve for the Unknown X and self-check your answers to see if your answer balances the equation.

a) 10 mg + 8 mg = X mg + 15 mg

b) X mL + 72.5 mL = 23.6 mL + 86.76 mL

c) 0.3 g + X g = 1.06 g + 0.05 g + 0.105 g

d) 23 1/4 tablets + 6 1/2 tablets = X tablets + 18 3/4 tablets

e) 17.6 mg – 7.3 mg = 14.8 mg – X mg

f) 1.2 mL – X mL = 0.8 mL – 0.15 mL

g) 6 1/4 tablet – X tablets = 10 3/8 tablets – 5 1/4 tablets

h) X mg – 23 mg = 35.6 mg – 12.7 mg

i) 3.15 mL + 4.37 mL = 8.65 mL – X mL

j) X g – 0.12 g = 1.07 g – 0.38 g

SECTION II
FINDING THE VALUE OF UNKNOWN X IN MULTIPLICATION AND DIVISION

The vast majority of dosage calculations require the veterinary professional to solve for the Unknown X in a multiplication or division type of problem. Therefore, being able to apply the basic algebraic rules to accurately isolate the Unknown X to one side is essential for solving dosage calculations problems.

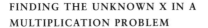
FINDING THE UNKNOWN X IN A MULTIPLICATION PROBLEM

If given three known values, the mathematical relationships between the known values, and then asked to find a fourth, Unknown value, we essentially follow the same steps that we did with the addition and subtraction problems.

1. Rearrange the equation, if necessary, to make the Unknown X a *positive* value.

2. Isolate the positive Unknown X on one side of the equation.

3. Perform the mathematical operation on the rearranged equation.

Let's illustrate this process with an example.

Mrs. Smith's dog has been on a single, 100 mg tablet daily. She prefers giving her dog smaller-sized tablets, so the veterinarian has written orders to dispense a bottle of 50 mg tablets at the dose of 2 tablets once daily. Previously she had been dispensed 35 of the 100 mg tablets (35 days worth of medication). How many 50 mg tablets will you need to dispense to give Mrs. Smith 35 days worth of medication?

One way of setting this problem up to determine the number of tablets needed would be as follows:

$$100 \text{ mg} \times 35 \text{ tablets} = 50 \text{ mg} \times X \text{ tablets}$$

Notice how one set of conditions (the original size and number of tablets) is set up on the left side of the equal sign, and the other set of conditions (the new size and Unknown number of tablets) is set up on the other side. Both conditions must equal each other because Mrs. Smith is counting on getting the exact same amount of medication, just in a different form.

As we mentally run through our checklist for solving this problem, the first question we ask is: "Is the Unknown X a positive number in the equation as we have written it?" The answer is "yes," so we proceed to step number two: isolate the Unknown X on one side of the equation.

Instead of subtracting or adding a value to the 50 mg to remove it from one side and put it on the other side of the equation, we take advantage of the multiplication law that says "Any value times 1 equals that value." In other words, we want to convert 50 mg to a value of 1 so that "1 × X" will equal X and will isolate the Unknown X on the right side of the equation by itself.

To convert 50 mg to 1, we multiply the 50 by its reciprocal (1 over 50). Any number multiplied by its reciprocal equals 1.

$$50 \times \frac{1}{50} = \frac{50}{50} = 1$$

When we multiply one side by the reciprocal of 50, we multiply the other side of the equation also because whatever we do to one side of the equation we have to do to the other side. When we do, we get something that looks like this:

$$100 \times 35 \times \frac{1}{50} = 50 \times \frac{1}{50} \times X$$

Now we can work the problem to find the answer for the Unknown X.

$$3500 \times \frac{1}{50} = 50 \times \frac{1}{50} \times X$$

$$\frac{3500}{50} = \frac{50}{50} \times X$$

$$70 = 1 \times X$$

$$70 = X$$

70 tablets are dispensed to give Mrs. Smith 35 days worth of medication.

Check it:

$$100 \times 35 = 50 \times X$$

$$100 \times 35 = 50 \times 70$$

$$3500 = 3500$$

Although the procedure looks more complex than the addition or subtraction procedures, it really is the same basic procedure. The two additional mathematical concepts used in these types of problems were

1. A number multiplied by its reciprocal equals 1.

2. Any value multiplied by 1 equals that value.

Below are two other examples. Notice that in the first example that the answer for the Unknown X was converted from a fraction to a decimal point, and in the second example the fraction of 1/10 has been replaced by the decimal equivalent of 0.1. Converting fractions to their decimal equivalents often makes for a simpler mathematical calculation.

Example:

$$0.25 \times 5 \times 8 = 2 \times 10 \times X$$

$$0.25 \times 40 = 20 \times X$$

$$10 = 20 \times X$$

$$10 \times \frac{1}{20} = 20 \times \frac{1}{20} \times X$$

$$\frac{10}{20} = \frac{20}{20} \ X$$

$$\frac{1}{2} = 1 \times X$$

$$\frac{1}{2} = X$$

$$0.5 = X$$

Check it:

$$0.25 \times 5 \times 8 = 2 \times X \times 10$$

$$0.25 \times 5 \times 8 = 2 \times 0.5 \times 10$$

$$0.25 \times 40 = 2 \times 5$$

$$10 = 10$$

Example:

$$X \times 10 = 25 \times 2$$

$$X \times 10 = 50$$

$$X \times 10 \times \frac{1}{10} = 50 \times \frac{1}{10}$$

$$X \times 10 \times 0.1 = 50 \times 0.1$$

$$X \times 1 = 50 \times 0.1$$

$$X = 5$$

Check it:

$$5 \times 10 = 25 \times 2$$

$$50 = 50$$

MULTIPLICATION PROBLEMS USING FRACTIONS AND MIXED NUMBERS

When encountering fractions in an Unknown X multiplication problem, we use the same basic techniques for isolating the Unknown X on one side of the equation.

$$2 \times 3 = \frac{3}{4} \times X$$

First we check to see if we need to move the Unknown X to make it positive. X is already shown as a positive number, so no move is necessary. Now, to isolate the Unknown X on the right side of the equation, we need to make 3/4 into a value of 1 by multiplying it and the other side of the equation by its reciprocal.

$$2 \times 3 \times \frac{4}{3} = \frac{3}{4} \times \frac{4}{3} \times X$$

$$6 \times \frac{4}{3} = 1 \times X$$

$$\frac{24}{3} = X$$

$$8 = X$$

Check it:

$$2 \times 3 = \frac{3}{4} \times 8$$

$$6 = \frac{24}{4}$$

$$6 = 6$$

For mixed numbers (whole numbers and fractions together), convert the mixed number into an improper fraction, then proceed as described for the previous problem.

$$3 \times 4 = 1\frac{1}{2} \times X$$

$$3 \times 4 = \frac{3}{2} \times X$$

($1\frac{1}{2}$ has been converted into $\frac{3}{2}$)

$$3 \times 4 \times \frac{2}{3} = \frac{3}{2} \times \frac{2}{3} \times X$$

$$12 \times \frac{2}{3} = 1 \times X$$

$$\frac{24}{3} = X$$

$$8 = X$$

FINDING THE UNKNOWN X IN A DIVISION PROBLEM

Division problems deviate somewhat from the essential steps used in the addition, subtraction, and multiplication problems shown previously. To isolate the Unknown X on one side of the equation, we need to remember these three basic mathematical rules.

1. The mathematical operation Number 1 ÷ Number 2 results in the same decimal answer as the fraction

Number 1
Number 2

therefore the two representations are equivalent.

2. The fraction $\dfrac{\text{Number 1}}{\text{Number 2}}$ can be converted to a decimal number form by dividing Number 1 (the numerator) by Number 2 (the denominator).

3. Any fraction with 1 in the denominator (the lower number) is equal to the value of the numerator (the upper number); so 3/1 = 3, 100/1 = 100, etc.

Let's use this example division problem and solve for the Unknown X.

$$45 \div 15 = X \div 25$$

Because of the first mathematical rule listed above, we can rewrite the problem as:

$$\frac{45}{15} = \frac{X}{25}$$

We know that we still have to isolate the Unknown X on one side of the equation and all the other known values on the other. In this problem we can see that we can turn the 1/25 value into the value of 1 by multiplying it by its reciprocal 25. Of course, we also have to multiply the other side of the equation by 25 to maintain the numerical balance of both sides of the equation.

$$\frac{45}{15} \times 25 = \frac{X}{25} \times 25$$

Now we can solve the problem as we would a typical multiplication Unknown X problem.

$$3 \times 25 = \frac{X}{25} \times 25$$

$$75 = X \times \frac{1}{25} \times 25$$

$$\left(\text{remember } \frac{X}{25} \text{ is the same as } \frac{1}{25} \times X \right)$$

$$75 = X \times 1$$

$$75 = X$$

Check it:

$$45 \div 15 = X \div 25$$

$$45 \div 15 = 75 \div 25$$

$$3 = 3$$

On occasions, when we convert from the "÷" format to the fraction format, the Unknown X ends up as a denominator (it is on the bottom). For example:

$$20 \div 5 = 36 \div X$$

$$\frac{20}{5} = \frac{36}{X}$$

If we move the 36 to the other side of the equation, we would have our known values set up to calculate the value for 1/X instead of the value of X! You know right away that this would result in an incorrect answer because we know, for example, that 1/2 is not the same as 2!

Therefore, this problem needs to be set up so that not only is the Unknown X on one side of the equal sign and all the known values on the other side, but the X must be in the *numerator* position; that is, it must be the top number.

In situations where we start out with the Unknown X in the denominator position, we need to "move" the Unknown X to the other side of the equation before doing the mathematical operation to solve Unknown X. In so doing, this will place the Unknown X value in the numerator position on the other side of the equation. In order to move X to the other side, multiply both sides of the equation by the reciprocal of 1/X (which would be X).

$$\frac{20}{5} = \frac{36}{X}$$

$$\frac{20}{5} \times X = \frac{36}{X} \times X$$

$$\frac{20}{5} \times X = 36 \times \frac{1}{X} \times X$$

$$\frac{20}{5} \times X = 36 \times 1$$

$$\frac{20}{5} \times X = 36$$

Now that we have the X in the numerator position, we need to isolate the Unknown X on one side of the equation. To move the values and isolate Unknown X, we multiply both sides by the reciprocal of the number we want to move.

$$\frac{20}{5} \times X = 36$$

$$\frac{20}{5} \times \frac{5}{20} \times X = 36 \times \frac{5}{20}$$

$$1 \times X = 36 \times \frac{5}{20}$$

$$X = \frac{180}{20}$$

$$X = 9$$

Check it :

$$20 \div 5 = 36 \div X$$

$$20 \div 5 = 36 \div 9$$

$$4 = 4$$

Whereas in the addition, subtraction,

and multiplication problems we checked to see if the Unknown X was positive, for division problems we always check to see if the Unknown X is in the numerator. If it isn't, the X must be moved to the other side of the equation before it is isolated.

UNKNOWN X PROBLEMS INVOLVING DIVISION OF FRACTIONS

What about circumstances in which a fraction is involved in the division problem?

$$30 \div 5 = X \div \frac{1}{2}$$

$$\frac{30}{5} = \frac{X}{\frac{1}{2}}$$

First check to see if the Unknown X value is in the numerator. It is, so we can proceed to isolate the Unknown X on the right side of the equation.

Perhaps the best thing to do with fractions in these situations is to use their decimal equivalents. The decimal equivalent for a fraction is always obtained by dividing the numerator by the denominator. Therefore, 1 divided by 2, as in the fraction 1/2, is equivalent to 0.5. Although it may look a little odd, go ahead and plug the decimal number into the problem.

$$\frac{30}{5} = \frac{X}{\frac{1}{2}}$$

$$\frac{30}{5} = \frac{X}{0.5}$$

The principles for isolating Unknown X are the same as the previous problems.

$$\frac{30}{5} \times 0.5 = \frac{X}{0.5} \times 0.5$$

$$\frac{15}{5} = X$$

$$3 = X$$

Check it!

$$30 \div 5 = X \div \frac{1}{2}$$

$$30 \div 5 = 3 \div \frac{1}{2}$$

$$30 \div 5 = 3 \div 0.5$$

$$6 = 6$$

By mastering the mathematical principles by which the values on either side of the equation can legitimately be moved, and by following the essential steps related to isolation of Unknown X, the veterinary professional should be able to perform a wide variety of dosage calculations.

SECTION II
PRACTICE PROBLEMS
(Answers are at the end of the chapter.)

a) $2.5 \times 4.5 = X \times 2.25$

b) $\dfrac{1}{2} \times \dfrac{3}{4} = X \times \dfrac{7}{8}$

c) $\dfrac{7}{8} \times X = \dfrac{6}{9} \times \dfrac{5}{6}$

d) $\dfrac{16}{12} \times \dfrac{2}{3} = \dfrac{24}{15} \times X$

e) $1\dfrac{2}{3} \times 3\dfrac{1}{6} = X \times 5\dfrac{1}{12}$

f) $6.5 \div 4.2 = X \div 3.8$

g) $\dfrac{3}{4} \div \dfrac{1}{2} = X \div \dfrac{5}{8}$

h) $\dfrac{18}{24} \div X = \dfrac{9}{32} \div \dfrac{1}{16}$

i) $\dfrac{96}{32} \div \dfrac{3}{2} = \dfrac{24}{18} \div X$

j) $2\dfrac{1}{4} \div 1\dfrac{1}{8} = X \div 3\dfrac{1}{16}$

ANSWERS FOR PRACTICE PROBLEMS

SECTION I

a) 3 mg	b) 37.86 mL
c) 0.915 g	d) 11 tablets
e) 4.5 mg	f) 0.55 mL
g) $1\dfrac{1}{8}$ tablets	h) 45.9 mg
i) 1.13 mL	j) 0.81 g

SECTION II

a) 5

b) $\dfrac{24}{56} = \dfrac{3}{7} = 0.4286$

c) $\dfrac{240}{378} = \dfrac{120}{189} = 0.635$

d) $\dfrac{480}{864} = \dfrac{5}{9} = 0.5556$

e) $\dfrac{1140}{1098} = \dfrac{570}{549} = \dfrac{190}{183} = 1.03825$

f) 5.88

g) $\dfrac{30}{32} = \dfrac{15}{16} = 0.9375$

h) $\dfrac{1}{6} = 0.1667$

i) $\dfrac{2}{3} = 0.667$

j) $\dfrac{98}{16} = \dfrac{49}{8} = 6.125$

CHAPTER 5 PROBLEMS

1) Determine the Unknown X for each of the following problems.

   a) 100 mL + 250 mL = X mL + 300 mL

   b) 34 mg + X mg = 74 mg + 28 mg

   c) X L + 2.31 L = 7.09 L + 1.39 L

   d) 0.034 g + 0.002 g = 0.009 g + X g

   e) 45 gr − 7.5 gr = X gr − 37.5 gr

   f) 278 mg − 32.5 mg = 302.5 mg − X mg

   g) X gr − 15 gr = 90 gr − 37.5 gr

   h) 0.025 mcg − X mcg = 0.09 mcg − 0.0763 mcg

2) Determine the Unknown X for each of the following problems.

a) $X \times 15 = 45 \times 5$

b) $16 \times 4 = 32 \times X$

c) $34.21 \times X = 33.41 \times 1.23$

d) $0.032 \times 0.0093 = X \times 0.0174$

e) $\dfrac{1}{16} \times \dfrac{3}{32} = X \times \dfrac{7}{8}$

f) $\dfrac{9}{18} \times \dfrac{3}{27} = \dfrac{54}{63} \times X$

g) $1\dfrac{1}{4} \times X = 3\dfrac{3}{4} \times 2\dfrac{1}{2}$

h) $X \times 5\dfrac{13}{24} = 6\dfrac{35}{42} \times 4\dfrac{3}{16}$

i) $24 \div 6 = 16 \div X$

j) $3.57 \div X = 4.63 \div 2.7$

k) $0.98 \div 12 = X \div 16.5$

l) $X \div \dfrac{1}{2} = \dfrac{3}{4} \div \dfrac{1}{4}$

m) $\dfrac{4}{15} \div \dfrac{4}{5} = \dfrac{9}{10} \div X$

n) $2 \dfrac{2}{3} \div X = 5 \dfrac{5}{12} \div 4 \dfrac{7}{8}$

3) A pharmacist puts 3 mL of one liquid in a graduated cylinder, to which he adds 12 mL of another liquid. If the pharmacist adds 5.75 mL to another graduated cylinder, how much of a second liquid would he have to add to the second graduated cylinder to equal the volume of the two liquids in the first graduated cylinder?

4) The veterinarian decides to use 3/4 of an ampule containing 240 mg of drug in a patient. If the veterinarian wanted to use an ampule containing 360 mg of the drug instead, what fraction of the 360 mg ampule would need to be used to provide the same dose?

5) A veterinarian determines that the total dose of phenobarbital for an epileptic dog is a combination of 7.5 mg tablet and 45 mg tablet. If she decides to use a 15 mg tablet in place of the 7.5 mg tablet, how much additional phenobarbital (in milligrams) will she need to give to create an equivalent dose?

MEASUREMENTS USED IN VETERINARY MEDICINE

Objectives

The student will be able to perform the following:

1. Define a given metric unit relative to other metric units of measure (e.g., grams compared to kilograms, etc.).
2. Convert simple key metric conversions to apothecary, household, or avoirdupois measurements used in veterinary medicine.
3. Recognize the symbols used for metric, apothecary, household, or avoirdupois measurements commonly used in veterinary medicine.

The units of length, volume and mass (weight) that we use every day are sometimes cumbersome to use in the medical area. Therefore, units of measurement in the medical field are often expressed as metric units (e.g., kilograms, milliliters, or centimeters). Other unit systems besides the metric system are also used. These include apothecary units (e.g., grains, drams), household units (e.g., teaspoons, cups), and avoirdupois units (ounces, pounds). To add to the confusion, each type of measurement system has its own values for length (e.g., meter, foot, etc.), volume (e.g., liter, gallon, dram, etc.), and mass or weight (e.g., gram, pound, grain).

In veterinary medicine we commonly use a more restricted number of units than may be found in human hospitals and pharmacies. However, it is important that the veterinary professional become very familiar with the proper use of these measurement systems used in veterinary medicine, how to convert between units within each system and between different measurement systems.

SECTION I METRIC UNITS

The metric system is widely used in medical and scientific fields across the world because of its simplicity. Although it is not necessary for you to understand all components of the metric system, it is important to understand how the system is set up and how to convert between different units within the metric system.

THE BASICS OF THE METRIC SYSTEM

The metric system contains three key elements: the meter for length, the liter for volume, and the gram for mass. All other variations of these three key elements are some power of 10 (e.g., 10, 100, 1/10, 1/1000, etc.). To what degree a given unit deviates from the basic measurement by a power of 10 is defined by the prefix. For example, the prefix *kilo* means to multiply the basic unit by 1000. Therefore:

1 kilogram	=	1000 grams
1 kilometer	=	1000 meters
1 kiloliter	=	1000 liters

The basic prefixes used in the metric system are:

kilo	multiplies by 1000	$\times 10^3$
hecto	multiplies by 100	$\times 10^2$
deka	multiplies by 10	$\times 10$
deci	multiplies by 1/10	$\times 10^{-1}$
centi	multiplies by 1/100	$\times 10^{-2}$
milli	multiplies by 1/1000	$\times 10^{-3}$
micro	multiplies by 1/1,000,000	$\times 10^{-6}$
nano	multiplies by 1/1,000,000,000	$\times 10^{-9}$

The prefixes most commonly used in veterinary medicine include *kilo-, centi-, milli-,* and *micro-. Deci-* is used in laboratory results such as glucose concentrations, blood urea nitrogen (BUN), and others. *Nano-* indicates a very small amount and is sometimes used in reporting drug concentrations within the body (e.g., digoxin). Of the prefixes most commonly used, only *kilo-* indicates an amount greater than the "base" unit (gram, liter, meter). All the other prefixes indicate a small, fractional amount. Therefore, in memorizing these units, remember that a kilo unit is the one that is larger than the base unit, and all the rest are smaller.

The metric prefixes all have specific abbreviations. The ones commonly used in veterinary medicine are shown below.

kilo	k
deci	d
centi	c
milli	m
micro	mc or μ (the Greek character mu)
nano	n

Note that when the Greek letter, μ, is handwritten, it can look very similar to a script *m* with pointed "peaks." Therefore, the *mc* designation is becoming more commonly used in handwritten dosing orders, although the μ is still often seen in typewritten text.

When referring to more than one metric unit (e.g., 300 kilograms), the abbreviation does not end with an *s*. Thus, 300 kilograms would be 300 kg, not 300 kgs.

METRIC UNITS OF WEIGHT OR MASS

The weight of a substance, such as the weight of an amount of drug or the weight of the patient, is expressed using the metric unit *gram* and adding the appropriate prefix. The metric prefixes commonly used with grams in veterinary medicine include:

kg	= kilogram	= 1000 grams	$=10^3$ grams
g	= gram		
mg	= milligram	= 1/1000 of a gram	$=10^{-3}$ grams
mcg	= microgram	= 1/1,000,000 of a gram	$=10^{-6}$ grams
μg	= microgram	= 1/1,000,000 of a gram	$=10^{-6}$ grams
ng	= nanogram	= 1/1,000,000,000 of a gram	$=10^{-9}$ grams

Notice how kilograms are 10^3 times (1000×) greater than grams, and milligrams are 10^{-3} times (0.001×) less than grams. Micrograms are an additional 10^{-3} (0.001×) smaller than milligrams, and nanograms are an additional 10^{-3} smaller than micrograms. Therefore, the major units of mass commonly used by veterinary professionals are conveniently spaced at intervals of 1000. Another way of saying this is that by moving the decimal point on a number three spaces to the right or left, you can easily convert from one unit value to another.

Note that older textbooks and publications may use the abbreviation for gram as *Gm*. This older expression is one of several that were in use prior to the standardization of abbreviations for the metric system in 1960. The *Gm* abbreviation for grams was used to differentiate from the apothecary measurement of mass called grains (gr). Today we use the lowercase letter *g* to represent the unit of gram and still use *gr* for grains.

In order to convert between the metric units for mass, there are certain conversions that the veterinary professional must either memorize or mathematically conceptualize. They are shown in the table below:

1 gram	=	1/1000 of a kilogram (kg)
1 milligram	=	1/1000 of a gram (g)
1 kilogram	=	1,000,000 milligrams
1 kilogram	=	1000 grams

Again, with these commonly used units, it is a matter of moving the decimal point three places right or left depending on whether the resulting number value is greater or less than the original value. The following examples show how one metric weight unit converts to another using these rules. In most cases it is simply a matter of moving the decimal to the right or to the left three places.

1 gram of phenylbutazone	= 1000 mg of phenylbutazone
23 gram mouse	= 0.023 kg mouse
5 kg cat	= 5000 g cat
230 mg of potassium bromide	= 0.23 g of potassium bromide

METRIC UNITS OF VOLUME

The metric units of volume are based on the unit of liters. The most common metric units of volume, their abbreviations, and their relationship to the base unit of liters are shown in the table below:

liter	= L			
milliliter	= mL	= 10^{-3} liter	=	0.001 liter
microliter	= mcL or μL	= 10^{-6} liter	=	0.000001 liter

Although other metric prefixes attached to liter are sometimes encountered, these are by far the most commonly used units in veterinary medicine.

Another unit of volume commonly used in medicine, especially oral and handwritten dosage orders, is "cc" or "cubic centimeter." Although centimeter is a unit of length, the volume described by a 1 cm × 1 cm × 1 cm cube is equivalent to 1 mL of volume. Therefore "cc" and "mL" are considered equivalent units.

Notice that the abbreviation for liter is L and not l. As you can tell by the text in this book, the lowercase l looks remarkably like the number 1. Therefore, to avoid confusion, the abbreviation for all liter measurements is listed as L.

Common relationships between units of volume that you should memorize are:

1 liter	=	1000 mL
1 liter	=	1000 cc
1 mL	=	1000 microliter (mcL or μL)
1 mL	=	1 cc

METRIC UNITS OF LENGTH

The basic unit of metric system length is the meter. To conceptualize how long a meter is, suffice it to say that it is slightly longer than the yard. The rules for converting between the meter and other metric units of length are the same for the metric units of volume and weight. The metric units of length most commonly used in veterinary medicine include:

kilometer	=	km	$= 10^3$ meters $=$	1000 meters
meter	=	m		
centimeter	=	cm	$= 10^{-2}$ meter $=$	0.01 meter
millimeter	=	mm	$= 10^{-3}$ meter $=$	0.001 meter
micrometer	=	mcm or μm $=$	10^{-6} meter $=$	0.000001 liter

The micrometer is also spoken or written as the *micron*. A rough rule of thumb (literally) for determination of the length of a centimeter can be seen by looking at the average person's thumbnail, which is approximately 2 cm across from side to side.

Common relationships that should be memorized include:

1 meter	=	100 centimeters
1 meter	=	1000 millimeters
1 centimeter	=	10 millimeters
1 kilometer	=	1000 meters

COMBINATION OF METRIC UNITS TO DESCRIBE DENSITY OR CONCENTRATIONS

Metric units are often combined to describe the density of an object or the concentration of a solute in a solution, such as the amount of drug that is dissolved in an amount of liquid. Concentrations of solutions are most commonly expressed as a unit of mass within a unit of volume. The following are concentrations and examples of how they might be used in veterinary medicine.

25 mg/cc (25 mg of dexamethasone in each cc of alcohol)

10 g/L (10 grams of disinfectant per liter of water)

0.5 kg/100 mL (0.5 or one-half kilogram per 100 mL of propylene glycol)

In large animal medicine and nutrition, we may encounter a concentration expression that is a unit of mass per another unit of mass. The most commonly encountered concentration of this sort is found where the weight of substances is contained within a certain weight of feed. For example, the following are situations in which feed additives or toxicants in feed are quantitated using a mass/mass set of metric units.

100 g/kg (100 g of toxicant per kilogram of feed)

3 mg/100 g (3 mg of feed additive per 100 grams of feed)

0.01 mg/kg (0.01 mg of drug per kg of feed)

SECTION I
PRACTICE PROBLEMS
(Answers are at the end of the chapter.)

1) Write the abbreviations that would be used for each of the following:

a) twenty kilograms

_____

b) ten point three milliliters

_____

c) thirty-five cubic centimeters

_____

d) five and one-tenth milligrams

_____

e) thirty-four and two-hundredths grams

_____

f) twenty-six and forty-three thousandths liters_____

g) fifteen milligrams per kilogram

_____

h) zero point zero one four grams per liter_____

2) Convert the following metric measures:

a) 10 kg   =   _____ g

b) 2 L   =   _____ mL

c) 250 mL   =   _____ L

d) 75 cc   =   _____ mL

e) 1500 mg   =   _____ g

f) 120 cm   =   _____ m

g) 2.5 km   =   _____ m

h) 3876 mm   =   _____ cm

SECTION II
COMMONLY USED HOUSEHOLD, APOTHECARY, AND AVOIRDUPOIS UNITS

Before the metric system was developed, units of measurement were based upon common utensils (teaspoon, cup, etc.) or readily accessible measuring units (foot, rod, grain of wheat). The apothecary measurement system was adopted by physicians and those who compounded medications from herbs and other natural sources as a means for measuring components for creating early medications. This system has been largely phased out. The avoirdupois system is also a much older system and is the system associated with units of weight such as ounces and pounds. Some of these units are still used in veterinary medicine, but most have been replaced by the metric system. The household measurement system is still used in many OTC (over-the-counter) consumer preparations, therefore the veterinary professional is likely to encounter these units in preparing some medications for dispensing.

Even though many of these units have been replaced by the metric system, it is important that the veterinary professional be able to recognize nonmetric system abbreviations, and be able to convert them to the metric system for dosage calculation.

COMMON UNITS

The following units are most commonly used in veterinary medicine. Their abbreviations and their metric equivalents are listed next to them.

Weight

| 2.2 pound | = 2.2 lb | = | 1 kg |
| 1 grain | = 1 gr | = | 60 or ~64 mg |

Volume

1 teaspoon	= 1 t or tsp	=	5 mL
60 drops	= 60 gtt	=	5 mL
1 tablespoon	= 1 T or tbs or Tbs	=	15 mL
1 ounce	= 1 oz	=	30 mL
1 cup	= 1 c	=	240 mL
1 pint	= 1 pt	=	480 mL
1 quart	= 1 qt	=	960 mL
1 gallon	= 1 gal	=	3.84 L

Note that the measurement for grain is
either 60 mg or approximately 64 mg. Both
conversions are still in use in describing the
amounts of medication found in tablets.
Different types of medication list 5 grains
as 300 mg or 325 mg. In most cases, where
medication is listed by grains, the metric
equivalent is also listed on the bottle or
container. Because the measurement of
grains is imprecise, it is avoided whenever
possible. Still, medications like phenobarbital and aspirin are commonly listed in grain
units. Therefore, it is important for the veterinary professional to be familiar with
both forms of metric equivalents of grain
units and to always check the bottle or container to identify which use of the grain

unit applies to the medication.

The veterinary professional may occasionally encounter, a dose in grains written as the apothecary notation gr 11/2 instead of 11/2 gr. Standard use in most of the veterinary literature uses the numerical value first followed by the unit gr.

The use of the single-letter abbreviations for tablespoon (T) and teaspoon (t) should be avoided in handwritten instructions or records because of the common confusion in identifying whether a handwritten *t* is an uppercase or lowercase letter. Because 3 teaspoons is equivalent to 1 tablespoon, there is a potential for a significant miscalculation of dose if the unit for teaspoon is read as tablespoon or vice versa.

Although the abbreviation for tablespoon is listed in some sources as *tbs* and *Tbs*, the more common usage is the form with the capitalized first letter *Tbs*.

CONVERSIONS BETWEEN COMMON HOUSEHOLD MEASUREMENTS

Because many of us have used household measurements and may be familiar with how a pint relates to a quart or a gallon, memorizing one conversion from household measurement to metric measurement can allow us to make the other conversions to metric from other household measurements. For example, if we memorize that 1 tablespoon is equivalent to 15 mL, and if we know the information in the table below, we can calculate the other metric equivalents for household measurements.

1 tablespoon	=	3 teaspoons
1 ounce	=	2 tablespoons
1 cup	=	8 ounces
1 pint	=	2 cups = 16 ounces
1 quart	=	2 pints = 4 cups = 32 ounces
1 gallon	=	4 quarts = 8 pints

If 1 tablespoon is equivalent to 15 mL, then 1 ounce must equal 30 mL (2×15 mL), 1 cup must equal 240 mL ($2 \times 8 \times 15$ mL), and 1 pint must equal 480 mL ($2 \times 8 \times 2 \times 15$ mL). Because dosages are listed in metric units and drugs or other compounds are sometimes listed as household volumes, the veterinary professional needs to be able to convert between household units and the metric system.

SECTION II
PRACTICE PROBLEMS
(Answers are at the end of the chapter.)

1) Write the abbreviations that would be used for each of the following:

a) twenty pounds

_____

b) ten point three grains

_____

c) thirty-five teaspoons

_____

d) five and one-half tablespoons

_____

e) three point two five ounces

_____

f) six and one-third cup

_____

g) fifteen gallons

_____

h) zero point five quart

_____

2) Convert the following measures:

a) 2 tsp   =   _____ mL

b) 2 Tbs   =   _____ mL

c) 150 mL   =   _____ Tbs

d) 30 mg   =   _____ gr

e) 4.4 lb   =   _____ kg

f) 3 kg   =   _____ lb

g) 3 gr   =   _____ mg

h) 45 mL   =   _____ tsp

SECTION III CONVERTING BETWEEN METRIC AND NONMETRIC MEASUREMENTS

Because medications, compounds, and delivery systems (e.g., syringes, bags of intravenous fluids) may come in metric or nonmetric units of measurement, the key equivalents should be memorized in order to facilitate making the conversions. We will focus on the conversions most commonly used in veterinary medicine.

THE COMMON EQUIVALENTS

Most of the conversions used in veterinary medicine involve converting between the metric system and the other systems of measurement. The following table shows the ones the veterinary professional should commit to memory:

1 kilogram	=	2.2 pounds
1 teaspoon	=	5 mL
1 tablespoon	=	15 mL
1 grain	=	60 mg

The one conversion commonly confused is the kilogram to pounds. A simple way to keep this in mind is to find your own weight in kilograms. Because 2.2 pounds equals only 1 kilogram, you should find that you are much "slimmer" when your weight is expressed in kilograms. For example, a 220 pound football linebacker becomes a 100 kilogram "weakling" when his weight is converted to the metric system. It is important to keep this relationship in mind so that you can check your answer mentally to see if the increase or decrease in numerical value of your answer makes sense. Try these examples and decide which of the two alternatives is the correct answer.

Does a 40 lb dog weigh 18.2 kilograms or 88 kilograms?

Does a 20 kg dog weigh 9.1 pounds or 44 pounds?

These conversions will be used in the next section to show you how to change between units.

SETTING UP A PROBLEM TO CONVERT FROM ONE UNIT TO ANOTHER

We can convert between many metric units by doing a mental calculation. However, in converting from nonmetric units to metric units (or vice versa), the conversions are not always so clean. Therefore, it is important to set up a system by which you calculate all conversions. By picking a method for calculating conversions that makes sense to you and using it all the time, you increase your consistency in producing the correct answer.

There are two methods that we will introduce at this point. They are often called by a variety of different names, but we will call them the proportion method and the cancel-out method. Algebraically they are very similar in their methodology, but they are set up slightly differently. Each method is equally reliable if you remember the rules for it. Pick one, become very familiar with it, and use it!

USING THE PROPORTION METHOD

Let's say we want to determine how many kilograms a 66 lb animal weighs. We need three things to set this problem up:

1) a given value in given units (66 lb)
2) the unit of the Unknown (kg)
3) a "conversion factor" (in this case, 2.2 lb = 1 kilogram)

The "conversion factor" is any equivalent equation in which the known and the Unknown units are involved. For example, we are converting pounds to kilograms, so we need to use a conversion factor that involves pounds and kilograms. The conversion of 1 kilogram = 2.2 pounds in the table above works nicely for this purpose.

To set the problem up, we set up a proportion of values on either side of an equation.

$$\frac{\text{UNKNOWN UNIT}}{\text{KNOWN VALUE UNIT}} =$$

$$\frac{\text{CONVERSION FACTOR WITH SAME UNITS AS UNKNOWN}}{\text{CONVERSION FACTOR WITH SAME UNITS AS KNOWN}}$$

For calculating how many kilograms a 66 pound animal weighs, we determine that the Unknown (X) value uses kilograms for its units.

$$\frac{X \text{ kg}}{?} = \frac{? \text{ units}}{? \text{ units}}$$

The known value in our problem is the 66 pounds. So we put that in the slot below the Unknown X:

$$\frac{X \text{ kg}}{66 \text{ lb}} = \frac{? \text{ units}}{? \text{ units}}$$

Finally set up the kilograms to pounds conversion factor so that similar units (kg or lb) are either both on the top or both on the bottom.

$$\frac{X \text{ kg}}{66 \text{ lb}} = \frac{1 \text{ kg}}{2.2 \text{ lb}}$$

We then solve for X by moving all the known values to the one side leaving the X kg alone on the other side of the equation. To do this, we multiply both sides of the equation by 66 to make the left side of the equation "X times 1," which is equivalent in value to X.

$$66 \text{ lb} \times \frac{X \text{ kg}}{66 \text{ lb}} = \frac{1 \text{ kg}}{2.2 \text{ lb}} \times 66 \text{ lb}$$

Any number times its reciprocal is equal to the value of 1. Therefore $66 \times 1/66 = 1$.

$$\frac{66 \text{ lb}}{66 \text{ lb}} \times X \text{ kg} = \frac{1 \text{ kg}}{2.2 \text{ lb}} \times 66 \text{ lb}$$

$$1 \times X \text{ kg} = \frac{1 \text{ kg}}{2.2 \text{ lb}} \times 66 \text{ lb}$$

$$X \text{ kg} = \frac{1 \text{ kg}}{2.2 \text{ lb}} \times 66 \text{ lb}$$

When we have similar units in the numerator and denominator on one side of the equation (such as the fraction of 66 lb over 66 lb), we were able to "cancel out" the unit of pounds. In effect, the pounds units in the numerator and denominator on the left side of the equation "disappeared," leaving just kilogram units on the Unknown side.

We can cancel out the pounds on the right side of the equation as well because there is a unit in pounds above the line (66 lb) and a unit of pounds below the line in the denominator of the fraction 1 kg/2.2 lb. Cancelling out the unit of pounds leaves only the kilogram unit on the right side of the equation. It is important that the units be the same on either side of the equation.

$$X \text{ kg} = \frac{1 \text{ kg}}{2.2 \cancel{\text{ lb}}} \times 66 \cancel{\text{ lb}}$$

$$X \text{ kg} = \frac{1 \text{ kg}}{2.2} \times 66$$

Now finish the calculation to find the value for X kg.

$$X \text{ kg} = \frac{1 \text{ kg}}{2.2} \times 66$$

$$X \text{ kg} = \frac{66 \text{ kg}}{2.2}$$

$$X \text{ kg} = 30 \text{ kg}$$

Check the answer by plugging the 30 kg into the equation to see if you arrive at the same numerical value on either side of the equal sign. Divide the numerator by denominator to find the decimal value for each side of the equation.

$$\frac{30}{66} = \frac{1}{2.2}$$

$$0.455 = 0.455$$

The answer of 30 kg is correct.

To repeat, we need to plug the known, the Unknown, and the conversion factor into the proportional equation below and solve.

$$\frac{\text{UNKNOWN UNIT}}{\text{KNOWN VALUE UNIT}} \quad =$$

$$\frac{\text{CONVERSION FACTOR WITH SAME UNITS AS UNKNOWN}}{\text{CONVERSION FACTOR WITH SAME UNITS AS KNOWN}}$$

Here is an example of using the proportional method to convert one metric unit to another.

How many kilograms are in a 340 gram bottle?

$$\frac{\text{X kg}}{340 \text{ grams}} = \frac{1 \text{ kg}}{1000 \text{ grams}}$$

$$340 \text{ g} \times \frac{\text{X kg}}{340 \text{ g}} = \frac{1 \text{ kg}}{1000 \text{ g}} \times 340 \text{ g}$$

$$\frac{340 \text{ g}}{340 \text{ g}} \times \text{X kg} = \frac{1 \text{ kg}}{1000 \text{ g}} \times 340 \text{ g}$$

$$1 \times X \text{ kg} = \frac{1 \text{ kg}}{1000} \times 340$$

$$X \text{ kg} = \frac{340 \text{ kg}}{1000}$$

$$X \text{ kg} = 0.34 \text{ kg}$$

Check it!

$$\frac{0.34}{340} = \frac{1}{1000}$$

$$0.001 = 0.001$$

Practice this method on the Practice Problems at the end of this section.

THE CANCEL-OUT METHOD

This method is sometimes called the "factor-label method," "unit conversion," or "dimensional analysis." By calling it the "cancel-out method," we are describing how this method works and is set up. No matter what name is used, the key to this method is to set up a multiplication problem so that all the units (mg, kg, mL, etc.) cancel each other out, leaving only the unit used for the Unknown.

To set up a problem in the cancel-out method, the Unknown is put on the left side of the equation, and then the known value and conversion factor are arranged into a multiplication problem on the right side of the equation so that the unit we wish to cancel out is present in both a numerator (top number in a fraction) and a denominator (bottom number) of the problem. The units in the numerator can then cancel out with an identical unit in the denominator.

To demonstrate this, let's use the same problem used on the proportion method above (How many kilograms is a 66 pound animal?). In that problem we have an Unknown X expressed in kilograms (kg), a known value of 66 lb, and a conversion factor of 2.2 lb = 1 kg. To set up the equation, first put the X with its units on the left side of the equation:

X kg =

On the other side of the equation, multiply the known value (66 lb) by the conversion factor set so that the known units (lb) cancel each other out leaving only the Unknown unit (kg) above the line in the numerator position.

$$X \text{ kg} = 66 \text{ lb} \times \frac{1 \text{ kg}}{2.2 \text{ lb}}$$

Now cancel out any units found both in the numerator and denominator.

$$X \text{ kg} = 66 \cancel{\text{ lb}} \times \frac{1 \text{ kg}}{2.2 \cancel{\text{ lb}}}$$

Canceling out the pounds leaves only units of kilograms on either side of the equation.

$$X \text{ kg} = 66 \times \frac{1 \text{ kg}}{2.2}$$

When we solve the calculation we get an answer in the units of the Unknown (kilograms).

$$X \text{ kg} = \frac{66 \text{ kg}}{2.2}$$

$$X \text{ kg} = 30 \text{ kg}$$

An advantage of the cancel-out method is that there is only *one* way you can set the right side of the equation up so that the pound (lb) units cancel leaving the kg above the line. If we had set up the equation improperly and multiplied the answer through, the resulting units would have looked rather peculiar:

$$X \text{ kg} = 66 \text{ lb} \times \frac{2.2 \text{ lb}}{1 \text{ kg}}$$

$$X \text{ kg} = \frac{145.2 \text{ lb}^2}{\text{Kg}}$$

(the lb² comes from lb × lb)

If the conversion factors are memorized and the rule for the cancel-out method is followed, you won't always have to remember whether to divide or multiply by 2.2 to convert pounds to kilograms or vice versa.

Below is the other example using the cancel-out method. Remember, the key is to set up the multiplication problem so that the known units cancel out leaving only the Unknown unit on one side of the equation.

How many kg in a 340 gram bottle?

The conversion factor used in this problem is 1 kilogram = 1000 gram. We are trying to find the number of kilograms. Set up the problem to cancel out grams and leave only kilograms.

$$X \text{ kg} = 340 \text{ g} \times \frac{1 \text{ kg}}{1000 \text{ g}}$$

$$X \text{ kg} = 340 \cancel{\text{g}} \times \frac{1 \text{ kg}}{1000 \cancel{\text{g}}}$$

$$X \text{ kg} = \frac{340 \text{ kg}}{1000}$$

$$X \text{ kg} = 0.34 \text{ kg}$$

It is important that you pick one method (proportion or cancel-out) that works best for you and practice it repeatedly to be able to consistently make these conversions when solving dosing calculations.

SECTION III
PRACTICE PROBLEMS
(Answers are at the end of the chapter.)

1) Calculate the following conversions:

a) 88 lb = _____ kg

b) 425 kg = _____ lb

c) 0.5 kg = _____ lb

d) 115 lb = _____ kg = _____ g

e) 325 tsp = _____ mL = _____ L

f) 56.75 Tbs = _____ mL = _____ L

g) 0.25 lb = _____ kg = _____ g

h) 0.00056 lb = _____ g (note the units!)

2) Find the weight in pounds for the following animals:

a) 25 kg dog _____

b) 5 kg cat _____

c) 453 kg horse _____

d) 145 kg pig _____

e) 74 kg person _____

f) 0.5 kg rat _____

3) Word problems; find the answer.

a) What is the combined total weight in kilograms of a 35 lb dog and a 9 lb cat?

b) How many pounds less does a 210 kg pony weigh than a 450 kg horse?

c) What is the difference in weight between a 35 lb dog and a 35 kg dog? Which weighs more?

d) A 45 kg dog had a hemangiosarcoma (type of large tumor) removed that weighed 4.5 pounds. How much did the 45 kg dog weigh (in kilograms and in pounds) after removal of the tumor?

e) A dog with congestive heart failure is retaining fluids. The weight has increased from 45 pounds to 25 kilograms. How much weight in kilograms and pounds did this dog gain?

ANSWERS FOR PRACTICE PROBLEMS

SECTION I

1) a) 20 kg   e) 34.02 g

   b) 10.3 mL   f) 26.043 L

   c) 35 cc   g) 15 mg/kg

   d) 5.1 mg   h) 0.014 g/L

2) a) 10,000 g   e) 1.5 g

   b) 2000 mL   f) 1.2 m

   c) 0.25 L   g) 2500 m

   d) 75 mL   h) 387.6 cm

SECTION II

1) a) 20 lb   e) 3.25 oz

   b) 10.3 gr   f) $6\frac{1}{3}$ c

   c) 35 tsp   g) 15 gal

   d) $5\frac{1}{2}$ or 5.5 Tbs   h) 0.5 qt

2) a) 10 mL   e) 2 kg

b) 30 mL

f) 6.6 lb

c) 10 Tbs

g) 180 mg
(or 195 mg)

d) 0.5 or $\frac{1}{2}$ gr (grain!)

h) 9 tsp

SECTION III

1) a) 40 kg

e) 1625 mL= 1.625 L

   b) 935 lb

f) 56.75 Tbs =
851.25 mL = 0.851 L

   c) 1.1 lb

g) 0.1136 kg = 113.6 g

   d) 52.3 kg =
52,300 g

h) 0.255 g

2) a) 55 lb

d) 319 lb

   b) 11 lb

e) 162.8 lb

   c) 996.6 lb

f) 1.1 lb

3) a) 20 kg

   b) 528 lb

   c) 35 kg dog =
77 lb, or a 42 lb difference

d) The dog weighed 42.95 kg or 94.5 lb after the tumor was removed.

e) 45 pounds = 20.45 kg,
   or an increase of 4.55 kg or 10 lb

CHAPTER 6 PROBLEMS

1. Make the following conversions:

a) 340 mg   = _____ g

b) 0.325 kg = _____ g   = _____ mg

c) 52 mL   = _____ cc   = _____ L

d) 0.0251 L = _____ mL

e) 3 km   = _____ m

f) 40 cm   = _____ mm = _____ m

g) 0.355 m = _____ cm   = _____ mm

h) 0.0003 kg = _____ mg

2. Make the following conversions between metric and nonmetric units.

a) 55 lb   = _____ kg

b) 20 kg   = _____ lb

c) 4 tsp   = _____ mL   = _____ L

d) 25 Tbs   = _____ mL = _____ L

e) 60 gtt   = _____ mL = _____ L

f) 90 mL   = _____ tsp = _____ Tbs

g) 90 mg   = _____ gr = _____ g

h) 0.4 kg = _____ gr = _____ g = _____ lb

2. A dog with epilepsy is being treated with 1/4 gr phenobarbital every 12 hours. How many <u>mg</u> of phenobarbital is he receiving <u>per day</u>?

3. If an animal is supposed to receive 3 tsp daily of a prescribed elixir and the client only has a 3 cc syringe with which to administer the drug by mouth, how many syringefuls of medication are going to have to be administered with each dose?

4. You have been given orders to administer medication to an 850 lb cow. Unfortunately the dose listed in your drug formulary is in mg/kg of body weight. Therefore you must convert the 850 pounds to kilograms. How many kg does this cow weigh?

5. The concentration of feed additive is listed on the new container you just purchased as containing 100 mg of additive per kg of powder in which it is mixed. The amount listed on the old package of the feed additive produced by another manufacturer is 0.1 kg additive per kg of powder. Are the concentrations equivalent?

6. Mrs. Jones calls the veterinary hospital and says her dog has just consumed 15 of the 1/2 grain tablets of an OTC (over-the-counter) medication that were spilled on the floor. Doc looks up the drug and calculates what a potentially lethal dose would be for a dog the size of Mrs. Jones' pet. He determines that consuming 0.5 kg would produce a significant toxicosis and 0.75 kg is lethal for most animals of this size. How many kg of drug did this dog ingest? Is he likely to be showing signs of toxicosis or in danger of dying?

7. The amount of injectable anesthetic drawn up would safely anesthetize a 9 kg cat or a 5 kg dog. The patient to receive the anesthetic is a toy-breed dog weighing 4.5 lbs. Is this dose an overdose, an underdose, or just about right?

8. You have 35 mg of an analgesic/sedative injectable preanesthetic left in the bottle. This will provide analgesia and sedation for about 140 lb worth of animals. You are going to administer the medication to the following animals in order. At which animal are you going to not have enough drug? How many total kg of animal will you be able to anesthetize with the 35 mg of drug?

| Sam | weight | 23 kg |
| Bert | weight | 10 kg |

Lilly	weight	16.5 kg
Zamphire	weight	2.7 kg
Ignatz	weight	4.3 kg
Poindexter	weight	5.1 kg
Shubert	weight	4.2 kg
Wussbaby	weight	3.5 kg
Princess	weight	6.0 kg

DRUG ORDERS AND MEDICATION LABELS

Objectives

The student will be able to perform the following:

1. Identify the components of a dosage regimen either in written or in spoken form.
2. Accurately use the common abbreviations for dose intervals, routes of administration, and dose forms.
3. Read and accurately interpret a dose label and extract the information needed to calculate a dose, handle and store the medication properly, and double-check that the dose formulation is safe to use by the route of administration requested.

Unfortunately one of the most common errors that occur in the administration of drugs is not in calculating drug dosages, but in misunderstanding the written drug orders, not using the proper medication prescribed, or not using the correct concentration of drug. Most veterinary professionals with more than a few years of experience have likely witnessed all of these occurring in the veterinary teaching hospital setting or in veterinary practice. In some cases the mistakes were caught before the medication was administered. In other situations the mistake was not detected until the animal began showing an adverse reaction to the medication or the dose administered.

Reading and questioning drug orders ensures that the proper medication is given. Writing clear and concise drug orders is also critical. And doing the "3-look procedure" when handling the medication is equally critical. The 3-look procedure means you:

1. Look at the medication bottle or container label when you pick it up.
2. Look at the medication bottle or container label as you are withdrawing drug from it.
3. Look at the medication bottle or container label when you put it down.

The 3-look technique has been effective in catching many, many errors before the drug was administered, and in some cases prevented fatal consequences.

To ensure patient safety, as well as the safety of the veterinary team and animal owner, it is essential that the veterinary professional develop the knowledge and skill to accurately write, read, interpret, and correctly carry out drug orders.

SECTION I THE DOSAGE REGIMEN

The dosage regimen has three components to it:

1. The amount of drug to be given (the dose)
2. The route by which the drug is to be given (intramuscular, intravenous)
3. How often the drug is to be given (the dose interval)

THE DOSE

The dose is the amount of the drug administered and is listed according to the drug's mass (e.g., mg, grams, etc.) for a particular animal or as the drug's mass per unit of body weight (e.g., mg drug/kg body weight) for any animal. For example, a reference text might list a *dose* for a drug as 10 mg/lb for any animal. But a 30 lb dog would have an administered *dose* of 300 mg of drug.

Instead of a single dose, some general doses for animals are listed as a *dose range*. In this case, the dose might be listed in a manner similar to the examples shown below:

1 to 3 mg / kg

10 to 15 mg / lb

0.5 to 1.0 g / kg

The veterinary professional can use any dose amount within the range for the dosage calculation. Dose ranges allow for adjustments in the calculated dose to accommodate the use of tablets or capsules that are not readily broken into halves.

Note that the dose is not listed according to volume (e.g., 5 mL, 0.1 L, etc.). The reason that volume, by itself, is not accurate for use as a dose amount is that drug bottles often come in different concentrations. For example, xylazine is a commonly used injectable sedative/analgesic drug. It comes in 20 mg/mL concentration form and 100 mg/mL concentration form. Therefore, 1 mL of the 20 mg/mL formulation would be a dose of 20 mg, whereas 1 mL of the 100 mg/mL form would be five times that dose amount (100 mg). Therefore, doses are usually listed in milligrams, grams, grains, or other units of mass.

On occasions, the dose may be listed as "1 tablet" or "2 capsules." This is legitimate only if the amount of drug in each tablet or capsule is also listed.

Correct: 100 mg ampicillin, 1 capsule every 8 hours

Incorrect: 1 tablet every 8 hours

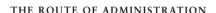
THE ROUTE OF ADMINISTRATION

The route of administration is the method by which a drug is introduced into the body. The common abbreviations used in veterinary medicine for routes of administration are listed below:

IM	intramuscular	injected into the muscle
IV	intravenous	injected into a vein
PO or po	per os	placed into the mouth and swallowed
SC or SQ	subcutaneous	injected just under the skin
ID	intradermal	injected into the skin
IP	intraperitoneal	injected into the peritoneal cavity
IA	intra-arterial	injected into an artery
PR	per rectum	placed within the rectum

Note that some sources prefer to use the abbreviations with periods between each letter (e.g., IM would be I.M.).

Drugs given by *parenteral* administration are given by injection somewhere between the intestinal tract and the surface of the skin (*para* = beside, *enteral* = GI tract). *Topically administered* drugs are those that are applied to the surface of the skin. Intravenous drugs can be given either as a single push or bolus, or administered over a period of time as an intravenous infusion.

■ Medical Mathematics and Dosage Calculations

Drugs given into the eye use the following abbreviations:

OS   left eye
OD   right eye
OU   each eye

Drugs given into the ear have a similar set of abbreviations:

AS   left ear (sometimes seen as AL)
AD   right ear
AU   each ear

THE DOSE INTERVAL

The dose interval is the amount of time between dose administrations, or the number of times a dose is administered within a given period of time (usually a day). The dose interval is usually abbreviated using the following standard notation.

q   every
h   hour
d   day
s.i.d.   once daily
b.i.d.   twice daily
t.i.d.   three times daily
q.i.d.   four times daily
q.o.d.   every other day (also
            abbreviated EOD, or q2d)
p.r.n.   as needed

STAT	immediately
qd	every day
q6h	every 6 hours
q8h	every 8 hours
q12h	every 12 hours

All of these abbreviations may be written in drug orders as uppercase (capitalized) letters, or with or without the periods.

Because some medication needs to be given with food to reduce GI side effects whereas other drugs need to be given when the stomach is empty to avoid problems with absorption, the following designations are used to denote when the drug should be given relative to a meal:

| ac | before meals |
| pc | after meals |

THE DOSE FORM

Sometimes the dose form is specified in the orders. The dose form of the medication can be solid, liquid, or gas. The common abbreviations used in veterinary medicine are shown below.

Solid dose forms:

tablet—tab
capsule—cap

Liquid dose forms:

> solution—sol
> suspension—susp
> elixir—elix
> tincture—tinct
> ointment—oint

Drug form descriptions may include "sustained release" or "controlled release." This refers to a particular type of tablet or capsule that releases the drug slowly over an extended period of time as the drug moves through the intestinal tract. Note that there are several drugs that come in both sustained release and regular release formulations. Because these different dose forms require different dosage regimens, it is important to note which formulation of drug is being ordered.

HANDLING UNCLEAR DRUG ORDERS

Unfortunately, written drug orders in a patient's record can sometimes be almost illegible. In these situations the primarily rule is *Do not guess what is written in the drug order; always confirm!* It is much easier to handle a simple question *before* the medication is given than to counteract an adverse drug reaction or overdose *after* the drug is administered!

SECTION I

PRACTICE PROBLEMS

(Answers are at the end of the chapter.)

1) For each of the following written orders, identify the drug, the dose, the dose interval, and the route of administration:

a) Give 50 mg of diphenhydramine by mouth three times a day.

b) Over the next 2 days I want this animal to get medicated every 12 hours with ampicillin. Give 300 mg and give it subcutaneously.

2) Translate the abbreviations for each of the following drug orders:

a) amoxicillin tabs 50 mg, 1 tab q8h PO

b) aspirin 125 gr PO prn

c) acepromazine 5 mg, 1 tab t.i.d. prn PO

d) neomycin oint, apply AU q6h for 7 d

e) tobramycin ophthalmic drops, 2 gtt q2h OD

f) methylprednisolone, 25 mg SQ q2d for 10 d

g) ampicillin, 120 mg b.i.d. IM

h) phenobarbital elix, 30 gr po qd pc

3) Write drug orders for each of the following using standard abbreviations:

a) Give 50 milligram Amoxi-Tabs® at the rate of three tablets twice daily for six days.

b) Administer one hundred twenty-five milligrams of azulfidine once daily as needed.

c) Place three drops of gentamicin in both eyes every four hours.

d) Inject 300 IU (international units) of penicillin G subcutaneously four times daily.

SECTION II MEDICATION LABELS

The medication label (which you should look at three times when dispensing medication!) contains critical information for carrying out drug orders. The label may also tell you important information about the nature of the drug, warnings for handling it, and how it should be stored.

THE DRUG NAME

On most drug containers (bottles, boxes, packages) there are usually two names listed for each drug. In the example shown in Figure 7.1, there is a capitalized name (Banamine) in large print with an R with a circle around it (®), and another name in parentheses below it in smaller font (flunixin meglumine).

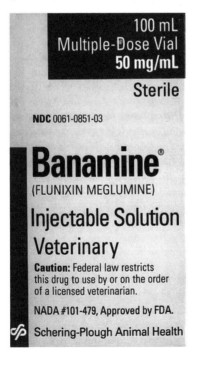

Figure 7.1 Banamine® (flunixin meglumine)

The name designated by the registered trademark ® or trademark ™ symbol is called the *proprietary* or *trade* name. The proprietary name is a proper noun (like Steve, Pam, etc.), and therefore it is capitalized. Banamine® and Amoxi-Tabs® would both be the trade names for the drug manufactured by a particular company. In most cases the trade name is the larger and more noticeable of the two names on the label because this name is the marketing name for the drug produced by the drug company. Another company manufacturing the exact same drug would have a different proprietary or trade name for its product. Therefore, for any given drug used in veterinary medicine, there may be two, three, or a dozen proprietary names for that drug.

The list below shows three different trade names (proprietary names) for a type of penicillin antibiotic called *amoxicillin*.

Amoxi-Tab®	=	amoxicillin tablets
Robamox-V®	=	amoxicillin tablets
Amoxil®	=	amoxicillin tablets

The smaller, second name on the label, written in lowercase letters, is called the *generic* or *nonproprietary* name, because it describes the drug itself and not that version of the drug produced by a particular manufacturing company. Unlike the proprietary name, the generic name is not capitalized because it is not a proper noun. In the list above, *amoxicillin* is the generic name for each of those drugs, and *flunixin meglumine* is the generic name for Banamine® in Figure 7.1. Because different pharmacies and veterinary hospitals will stock different proprietary named drugs from different manufacturers, using the *generic* or *nonproprietary* name reduces both confusion and the chance for making a mistake by using the wrong drug.

Certain trade names are so well recognized in veterinary medicine that they are widely used as a generic name to represent all drugs of that type. For example, the trade name Valium® is widely used in place of its generic name, diazepam. Because of this, it is important for the veterinary professional to recognize these widely used trade names and to know what their generic names are. Following are just a few of the more commonly used trade names in veterinary medicine.

```
Valium ®      = diazepam
Lasix ®       = furosemide
Tribrissen ® = sulfadiazine trimethoprim
Baytril ®     = enrofloxacin
LA 200 ®      = oxytetracycline
```

Most antiparasitic drugs and deworming medications are known by their trade names. New drugs released to the veterinary market are usually discussed in casual conversation by their highly publicized trade name. Because a new drug on the veterinary market is usually the only brand of its type available, people can get away with using the trade name for a time and be fairly accurate. However, it is still a good habit to refer to the drug by its generic name for accuracy when writing drug orders, recording drug administration in the patient record, or communicating with professional colleagues.

DOSE STRENGTH OR CONCENTRATION

As was pointed out previously, injectable drugs and tablets can come in different concentrations or amounts. Therefore, on each bottle, vial, or container of medication, there is a dosage strength or a concentration listed.

On the packaging for the injectable drug in Figure 7.2, the concentration of drug per volume of liquid is listed as 2 mg/mL. This tells us that for each mL we inject into the animal, we are delivering 2 mg of drug. Obviously a drug containing a more concentrated solution of drug, say 100 mg/mL, would deliver more drug with each mL injected.

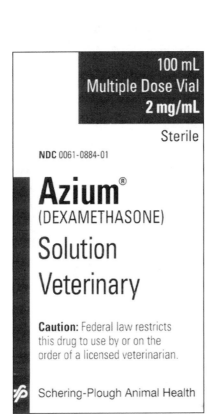

Figure 7.2 Azium® (dexamethasone)

DOSE STRENGTH LISTED AS A PERCENT SOLUTION

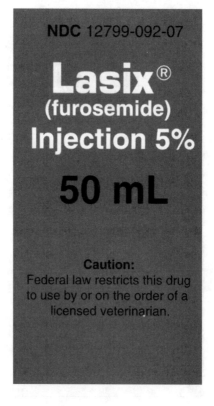

Figure 7.3 Lasix® (furosemide)

Notice on the drug above that the concentration of the drug in each mL is not listed as mg/mL. Instead the concentration is listed as a *percent solution* of 5%. The 5% means that there are 5 *grams* of drug in each *100* mL of liquid in this bottle. Therefore, a listing of X percentage solution means:

$$X\% = \frac{X \text{ grams}}{100 \text{ mL}}$$

To convert percentage solution to the more familiar mg/mL, divide the top and bottom of the gram/mL by 100, and then convert the grams into mg using the techniques previously described in Chapter 6 for converting between metric units.

$$5\% = \frac{5 \text{ grams}}{100 \text{ mL}} = \frac{0.05 \text{ grams}}{\text{mL}} = \frac{50 \text{ mg}}{\text{mL}}$$

Instead of memorizing the definition of percentage solution (X grams/100 mL), some students prefer to memorize the conversion for X percentage solution to mg/mL:

$$X\% = \frac{(X \text{ times } 10) \text{ mg}}{\text{mL}}$$

$$5\% = \frac{(5 \times 10) \text{ mg}}{\text{mL}}$$

$$5\% = \frac{50 \text{ mg}}{\text{mL}}$$

Either way, the definition or conversion for percentage solution must be memorized so that a drug listed as this type of concentration can be more easily used in dosage calculations.

Tablets and capsules also contain a "concentration" of sorts, but we usually refer to the amount of drug per tablet or capsule as the "strength." Therefore, the concentration or strength for solid dose forms might be 50 mg/tablet or 200 mg/capsule. Many times a given trade name comes in a variety of concentrations. For example, Amoxi-Tabs® comes in 50 mg, 100 mg, 200 mg, and 400 mg strengths.

DOSE FORMULATION AND NUMBER OF DOSE FORM UNITS

Notice on the florfenicol box shown in Figure 7.4 that the drug formulation was listed as an "injectable solution." Each drug package will state the formulation, or dose form, most commonly as a solution, suspension, tincture, elixir (all for liquid dose forms), tablets, or capsules (for solid dose forms). There are many variations from these basic dose forms including caplets, lozenges, and enteric-coated tablets.

The dose formulation does convey information about how the drug is to be used. For example, if the drug is listed as an elixir, it is taken internally (e.g., phenobarbital elixir for seizure control); but if it is a tincture, it is to be applied topically (e.g., iodine tincture for disinfection). A solution may be given intravenously, but a suspension is never given intravenously. An ointment melts at body temperature and so is

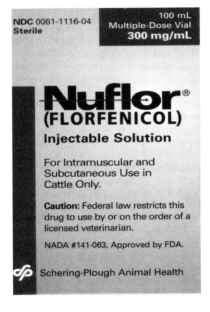

NDC 0061-1116-04
Sterile

100 mL
Multiple-Dose Vial
300 mg/mL

Nuflor®
(FLORFENICOL)

Injectable Solution

For Intramuscular and
Subcutaneous Use in
Cattle Only.

Caution: Federal law restricts this
drug to use by or on the order of a
licensed veterinarian.

NADA #141-063, Approved by FDA.

Schering-Plough Animal Health

Figure 7.4 Nuflor® (florfenicol)

usually applied topically (e.g., ointment for ear infections) whereas a paste retains its shape at body temperature and is more commonly used orally (e.g., equine deworming medications).

The dose formulation may also describe other characteristics that tell something about how a drug interacts with the body or how it should be used. For example, the "sustained release" formulation means that the drug will be given less frequently than a drug that is in a "regular" release formulation. A drug listed as an "enteric coated" tablet means that the drug doesn't begin to dissolve until it passes out of the stomach and into the intestine.

Injectable drugs whose dose form is described as a "vial" are usually small glass bottles with a rubber stopper that allows medication to be withdrawn with a needle several times. The exception to this would be the "single-dose vial" commonly used with vaccines. Ampules, on the other hand, are small glass bottles intended to be broken apart (usually snapped at a scored line on a narrow part of the ampule) and the contents used all at one time.

In addition to the dose form, the drug label lists the total number of units of the dose form contained within the package. For example, for the drug in Figure 7.4, the total volume of liquid drug in the bottle is listed as 100 mL. If this medication were in a tablet dose form, the total number of tablets in the bottle would be listed. Information about the total number of tablets can be critical information in determining the potential for toxicity if an ani-

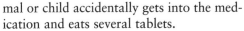
mal or child accidentally gets into the medication and eats several tablets.

Knowing the dose formulations and how they are used allows the veterinary professional to double-check the route of administration in the orders with the particular dose formulation that is being prescribed.

EXPIRATION DATES

All manufacturers of medications are required to list the expiration date on each container of drug. Obviously this date is intended to be a "discard this drug" date. In spite of the temptation to keep drugs on the veterinary hospital shelves beyond the expiration date for monetary reasons, the drugs should be discarded. At best, a drug will lose potency (strength) after the expiration date. In some circumstances, drugs break down in the container to a compound that may produce side effects or be toxic to the animal. Therefore, the safe and legal rule of thumb is that once a drug is beyond its expiration date, it should no longer be used on veterinary patients.

CONTROLLED SUBSTANCES LABELING

Substances that require special handling by law or for safety reasons have information displayed on the label that alerts the veterinary profession to those facts. For example, the package of meperidine shown in Figure 7.5 has a large capital C with a Roman numeral II prominently displayed.

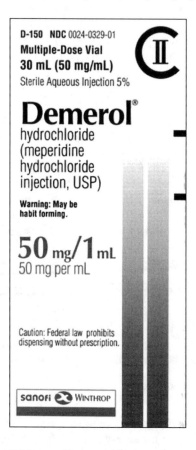

D-150 NDC 0024-0329-01

Multiple-Dose Vial
30 mL (50 mg/mL)
Sterile Aqueous Injection 5%

Demerol®
hydrochloride
(meperidine
hydrochloride
injection, USP)

**Warning: May be
habit forming.**

50 mg/1 mL
50 mg per mL

Caution: Federal law prohibits
dispensing without prescription.

sanofi 🞉 WINTHROP

Figure 7.5 Demerol® (meperidine)

The large *C* plus a Roman numeral II, III, IV, or V indicates that the drug is considered a *controlled substance* (a potentially abusive substance) and therefore requires special handling, record keeping, and storage of the drug based on which Roman numeral is listed. As a general rule, the lower the Roman numeral, the more potential for abuse the drug is considered to have and the greater the restrictions and record required. Therefore, a C-II drug, like Demerol® and other strong opioid narcotic agents, will have a much greater potential abuse than a C-IV drug like butorphanol. For further details on how controlled substances need to be stored and recorded, consult a textbook on pharmacy procedures or veterinary pharmacology.

USP AND NF LABEL DESIGNATIONS

Sometimes a drug package, like the acetaminophen tablets in Figure 7.6, will contain only a generic drug name and its dose formulation (in this case, tablets) followed by the initials *USP*. The acetaminophen shown was manufactured by a drug company that decided *not* to assign its own trade name to the drug and instead used the generic or nonproprietary name that is registered in the United States Pharmacopoeia. This often occurs when a drug is so widely manufactured that one particular trade name out of all the manufacturers' brands on the market is unlikely to be noticed (e.g., aspirin, acetaminophen, phenobarbital). Or sometimes a particular trade name is so well known in the market that it would not be beneficial for a competitor to market the drug under a different trade name. For example, many brands of diazepam are listed by the USP nonproprietary name because the name recognition of Valium® brand of diazepam is so strong.

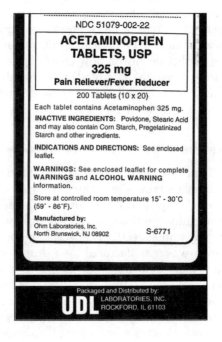

Figure 7.6 Acetaminophen

Other initials occasionally seen in place of USP are *NF*, which stands for the *National Formulary*. The National Formulary is another recognized standard similar to the United States Pharmacopoeia and is used on drug labels in basically the same manner.

HAZARD WARNINGS ON THE LABEL

If the drug poses a **potential health hazard** to the person administering the drug, a **potential hazard to the patient,** or other very important characteristics, a caution statement or warning statement will be found on the label. If the important information is rather detailed, the listing on the label will direct the reader to the "package insert" or the "prescribing information" that accompanies the container when it is shipped from the manufacturer. For example, the drug in Figure 7.7 warns the administrator of the drug to watch for a drop in blood pressure when the drug is injected.

Other warnings may include species restrictions ("For use in horses only" or "Not for use in horses intended for food"), cautions about route of administrations ("For oral use only," "For intravenous infusion only," "Restricted to topical use only"), abuse potential ("WARNING: May be habit forming"), or appearance of the drug ("Do not use if product is discolored").

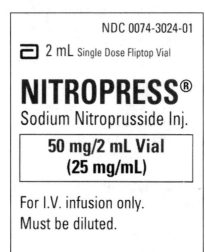

Figure 7.7 Nitropress® (sodium nitroprusside)

STORAGE INFORMATION ON THE LABEL

Often the package or label states information about how the drug should be stored. This information is often printed on one of the sides of the box, bottle, or drug container that is not on the front of the container. For example, on boxes of Baytril® (enrofloxacin) two statements sum up the key storage warnings: "Protect from direct sunlight. Do not freeze."

Storage information should be followed closely, as temperature fluctuations can change the physical form of the drug by either degrading the effectiveness of the drug or changing the absorption characteristics of the drug. For example, freezing and thawing injectable penicillin-G suspensions may change the crystal size of the drug, resulting in a drug that is much more painful when injected and absorbed more erratically. Drugs that are stored in the practice truck used by large animal and equine ambulatory veterinarians are especially susceptible to environmental exposure and storage conditions outside of the recommended range.

SECTION II
PRACTICE PROBLEMS
(Answers are at the end of the chapter.)

1) Answer the following questions from the information contained on the drug label in Figure 7.8:

   a) What is the trade name of this drug?

b) What is the generic or nonproprietary name of this drug?

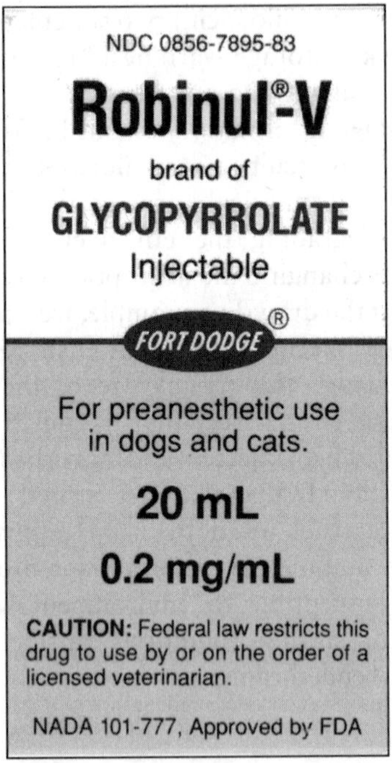

NDC 0856-7895-83

Robinul®-V

brand of

GLYCOPYRROLATE

Injectable

FORT DODGE ®

For preanesthetic use in dogs and cats.

20 mL

0.2 mg/mL

CAUTION: Federal law restricts this drug to use by or on the order of a licensed veterinarian.

NADA 101-777, Approved by FDA

Figure 7.8 Robinul®-V (glycopyrrolate)

c) How many mg of drug are in each milliliter of liquid?

d) How many 1 mL injections can you get from this bottle?

e) Is this a controlled substance? How
do you know?

f) What is the approved use for this
drug?

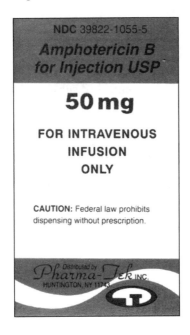

NDC 39822-1055-5

**Amphotericin B
for Injection USP**

50 mg

**FOR INTRAVENOUS
INFUSION
ONLY**

CAUTION: Federal law prohibits
dispensing without prescription.

Distributed by
Pharma-Tek INC.
HUNTINGTON, NY 11743

Figure 7.9 Amphotericin B USP

2) Answer the following questions from the
information contained on the drug label in
Figure 7.9:

a) Does this drug appear to have a trade

name? Explain how you determined this.

b) What is the generic or nonproprietary name of this drug? What does *USP* mean?

c) Can this drug be given intramuscularly?

d) Is this a controlled substance? How do you know?

3) List the following percentage solutions in the corresponding units.

a) 5%   = _____ g/100 mL

b) 0.3%   = _____ g/100 mL

c) 7.25%   = _____ mg/mL

d) 21.7%   = _____ mg/mL

e) 0.02%   = _____ mg/mL

ANSWERS FOR PRACTICE PROBLEMS

SECTION I

1) a) drug = diphenhydramine
      dose = 50 mg

dose interval = three times daily (t.i.d.)
route of administration = by mouth (PO)

b) drug = ampicillin
dose = 300 mg
dose interval = every 12 hours (q12h)
route of administration = subcutaneously (SQ)

2) a) Give one 50 milligram tablet of amoxicillin every eight hours by mouth.

b) Give 125 grains of aspirin by mouth as needed.

c) Give one 5 milligram tablet of acepromazine three times daily by mouth as needed.

d) Apply neomycin ointment into both ears every six hours. for seven days.

e) Give 2 drops of tobramycin ophthalmic drugs every two hours in the right eye.

f) Give 25 milligrams of methylprednisilone subcutaneously every two days (or every other day) for 10 days.

g) Give 120 milligrams of ampicillin intramuscularly twice daily.

h) Give 30 grains of phenobarbital elixir by mouth once daily after a meal.

3) a) Amoxicillin, 50 mg, 3 tabs b.i.d. (or q12h) 6d

b) azulfidine, 125 mg qd (or s.i.d.) prn

c) gentamicin, 3 gtt OU q4h

d) penicillin G, 300 IU SQ q.i.d. (or q6h)

SECTION II

1) a) Robinul®-V

b) glycopyrrolate

c) 0.2

d) 20

e) No. There is no C on the label.

f) Preanesthetic for dogs and cats

2) a) No. There isn't a ® or a ™ symbol by the drug name.

b) Amphotericin B. United States Pharmacopoeia

c) No. It is to be used for intravenous infusion only.

d) No. There is no C on the label.

3) a) 5%   =   5 g/100 mL

  b) 0.3%   =   0.3 g/100 mL

  c) 7.25% =   72.5 mg/mL

  d) 21.7% =   217 mg/mL

  e) 0.02% =   0.2 mg/mL

CHAPTER 7 PROBLEMS

1. Write the abbreviations for each of the following terms or phrases:

a) placed into the mouth and swallowed

_____

b) injected into an artery

_____

c) injected into the skin

_____

d) injected under the skin

_____

e) injected into the peritoneal cavity

_____

f) right eye   _____

g) left ear   _____

h) both eyes   _____

i) before meals   _____

j) after meals   _____

k) "every" (as in every three hours)

_____

l) immediately   _____

m) as needed   _____

n) solution   _____

o) ointment   _____

p) elixir   _____

2. Convert the following abbreviations into their indicated units (abbreviated):

a) q6h   =   __. i. d.

b) t.i.d.   =   q __ h

c) EOD   =   q __ d

d) q.i.d.   =   q __ h

e) q12h   =   __. i. d.

3. For each of the following, identify what is wrong with the abbreviations used in the drug and make the appropriate corrections.

a) Give 25 mg of ampicillin four times a day orally whenever it is needed.

ampicillin 25 g q4h prn

b) Inject 250 mg of amoxicillin under the skin every day for 10 days.

amoxicillin 250 gm b.i.d. 10h

c) Administer 2 drops of tobramycin in the right eye every 2 hours for one week.

tobraxin 2 gtts AD b.i.d. 7d

d) Apply DMSO topically four times daily as needed.

DMSO ID q4h PRN

e) Swallow 2 cimetidine tablets three times daily after each meal.

cimetidine caps q8h OP ac

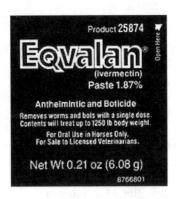

Figure 7.10 Eqvalan® (ivermectin)

4. For the drug in Figure 7.10, answer the following questions:

a) What is the dose form for this drug?

b) What is the concentration in mg/mL?

c) Can this drug be used in cattle?

5. For the drug in Figure 7.11, answer the following questions:

a) The word *Halothane* is capitalized. Is this the drug's trade name? Explain why or why not.

b) How is this drug to be stored? Is it okay to store it in the practice truck parked in an unheated garage on a cold December evening in Wisconsin?

c) What is the use for this drug?

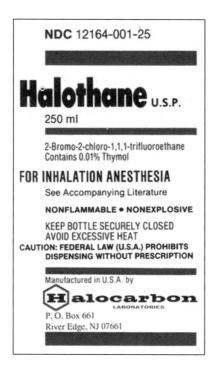

NDC 12164-001-25

Halothane U.S.P.

250 ml

2-Bromo-2-chloro-1,1,1-trifluoroethane
Contains 0.01% Thymol

FOR INHALATION ANESTHESIA

See Accompanying Literature

NONFLAMMABLE • NONEXPLOSIVE

KEEP BOTTLE SECURELY CLOSED
AVOID EXCESSIVE HEAT
CAUTION: FEDERAL LAW (U.S.A.) PROHIBITS
DISPENSING WITHOUT PRESCRIPTION

Manufactured in U.S.A. by

Halocarbon
LABORATORIES

P. O. Box 661
River Edge, NJ 07661

Figure 7.11 Halothane USP

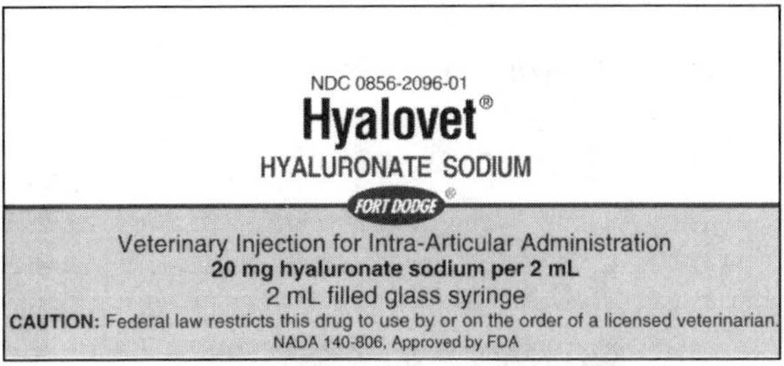

NDC 0856-2096-01

Hyalovet®

HYALURONATE SODIUM

FORT DODGE®

Veterinary Injection for Intra-Articular Administration
20 mg hyaluronate sodium per 2 mL
2 mL filled glass syringe
CAUTION: Federal law restricts this drug to use by or on the order of a licensed veterinarian.
NADA 140-806, Approved by FDA

Figure 7.12 Hyalovet® (hyaluronate sodium)

6. For the drug in Figure 7.12, answer the following questions.

a) When ordering the generic form of this drug, what name would you use?

b) What is unique about this dose form?

c) What is the total amount (mass) of drug in this package?

d) What is the concentration of drug in this package (mg/mL)?

7. For the drug in Figure 7.13, answer the following questions.

a) Isoflurane USP is listed on the box. Does this drug have a trade name?

b) Can this drug be used in all horses? Explain.

c) Can we determine the concentration of this drug from the label? Explain.

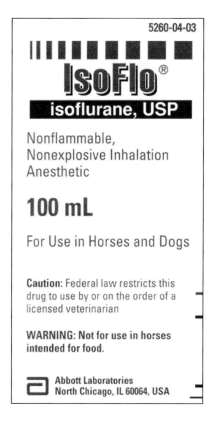

Figure 7.13 IsoFlo® (isoflurane, USP)

8. Think of the most intimidating personality you know. Now, let's say you have just

started working for this tyrant who also has a short fuse on his/her temper and doesnot hesitate to yell at anyone who he/she thinks might be the least bit incompetent. And he/she thinks almost everyone is incompetent, especially newcomers to the staff like you. He/she has just scribbled you a note with drug orders on it to be filled for a personal client who is waiting to pick up the medication. Your boss, the tyrant, is rushing out the door to his/her car when you look at the note and realize you can't really make out for certain the drug name. You have a pretty good idea of what it is (about a 70% chance of being correct), but the writing is poor enough that you can't tell for sure. The tyrant is late for a business appointment across town and obviously is in a hurry. Are you going to rush out the door after the tyrant/boss and risk being chewed out as an incompetent on your first day of work? How will you handle this? What alternatives will go through your mind?

DOSE CALCULATION AND SYRINGE MEASUREMENTS

Objectives

The student will be able to perform the following:

1. Convert an animal's weight from pounds to kilograms and vice versa.

2. Calculate the individual dose for an animal.

3. Determine the number of dose form units to administer to a given animal.

4. Determine the total number of dose form units to be dispensed over the span of a dosage regimen.

5. Read and interpret the markings on syringes in order to properly fill a syringe with the appropriate volume of drug.

Once the basic mathematical manipulations to find the Unknown X are understood and the components of the dosage regimen, including abbreviations, have been mastered, we can calculate the dose for the patient. In this section we will concentrate on the basic dose calculation method and then apply it to filling a hypodermic syringe with the appropriate amount of medication.

SECTION I THE BASIC DOSE CALCULATION

In calculating a dose, you always need three pieces of information:

1. The weight of the animal
2. The dose (amount of drug per weight of animal)
3. The concentration of the drug in the dose form (mg/mL, mg per tablet, etc.)

Although you may have to make some adjustments in the basic method for calculating the dose (e.g., converting the animal's weight from pounds to kilograms), once the three steps above are memorized and practiced, it should be relatively easy to calculate most dosages given in drug orders.

CONVERTING THE ANIMAL'S WEIGHT FOR DOSE CALCULATION

Typically the animal's weight is recorded in pounds and occasionally in metric units. Because most doses are listed in metric units (e.g., mg drug/kg body weight), it becomes necessary to convert the weight of the animal from pounds to units in the metric system.

In Chapter 6 we showed how to convert from nonmetric to metric units using the proportion method and the cancel-out method. As a quick review, we will illustrate how to convert a 44 lb dog's weight to its kilogram equivalent.

The proportion method sets up an equation as shown below where the known value unit is 44 pounds, the unknown unit is kilograms (kg), and the conversion factor is 2.2 lb = 1 kg.

$$\frac{\text{UNKNOWN UNIT}}{\text{KNOWN VALUE UNIT}} =$$

$$\frac{\text{CONVERSION FACTOR WITH SAME UNITS AS UNKNOWN}}{\text{CONVERSION FACTOR WITH SAME UNITS AS KNOWN}}$$

$$\frac{\text{X kilograms}}{44 \text{ lb}} = \frac{1 \text{ kilogram}}{2.2 \text{ lb}}$$

$$\text{X kg} = \frac{1 \text{kg} \times 44 \cancel{\text{lb}}}{2.2 \cancel{\text{lb}}}$$

$$\text{X kg} = 20 \text{ kg}$$

Check it:

$$\frac{20 \text{ kg}}{44 \text{ lb}} = \frac{1 \text{kg}}{2.2 \text{ lb}}$$

$$0.45 = 0.45$$

Both sides are equal so the answer was correct.

By the cancel-out method, we arrive at the same answer. Remember in the cancel-out method we put the Unknown X on one side and all the other values on the other side of the equation in such a way that all units (in this problem, pounds) cancel out leaving only the unit of the unknown (kilograms).

UNKNOWN UNIT = KNOWN VALUE ×

CONVERSION FACTOR WITH SAME UNITS AS UNKNOWN
CONVERSION FACTOR WITH SAME UNITS AS KNOWN

$$X \text{ kg} = 44 \text{ lb} \times \frac{1 \text{kg}}{2.2 \text{ lb}}$$

$$X \text{ kg} = \frac{44 \text{ kg}}{2.2}$$

$$X \text{ kg} = 20 \text{ kg}$$

Again, remember that either method of calculation arrives at the same answer, and it is up to each individual to decide which method is more comfortable.

TYPES OF DOSES LISTED

The dose for a given drug will be listed either in a formulary, a drug compendium book such as the *Veterinary Drug Handbook* by Donald Plumb, or on the package itself. The drug in most cases will be listed as an amount (mass) of drug per unit of body weight:

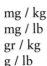
mg / kg
mg / lb
gr / kg
g / lb

In some instances drugs are listed in "absolute" values instead of per unit of body weight. For example, this dose for the estrogen compound diethylstilbestrol (DES) is listed as

0.1 to 1 mg PO daily for 3–5 days

Note that if you were to give 1 mg *per kilogram* of body weight of DES that the animal would be grossly overdosed! Therefore clinicians will sometimes circle or underline a dose like this to emphasize that it is not based on a per unit body weight like most dosages.

Occasionally some medications, like chemotherapeutic agents (for treating cancer) and digoxin (a cardiac medication), are listed according to *body surface area* instead of weight.

Digoxin: 0.22 mg/m^2 where m^2 is *meters square*, a measure of surface area

The thought behind this method of listing a dose is that at the extreme ends of the size, very small animals may receive too little drug if dosed on a mg/kg basis, and very large animals may receive too much drug. The body surface area can be converted to kilograms of body weight, and vice versa, using tables found in veterinary pharmacology books or veterinary drug formularies.

Remember that some doses are listed as a dose range instead of one amount of drug per unit of body weight. This allows the veterinary professional to adjust the dose to the available dose form. For example, if a dose range is 2 to 3 mg/lb, a 10 pound animal can receive any dose between 20 to 30 mg. If our tablet sizes for this drug come in 10 mg, 25 mg, and 50 mg sizes, the dose range allows us to select a dose form that would be most convenient for the owner or client to use in their animal (e.g., using a whole tablet instead of having to cut a tablet in half).

DETERMINING THE AMOUNT OF DRUG FOR A PARTICULAR ANIMAL

Given the body weight and the dose per unit of body weight, we can calculate the dose for the particular animal using either the proportional method or the cancel-out method. The Unknown X that we are calculating is the amount of drug (mg, g, gr, etc.) to be given to the animal. The known element in this problem is the body weight, and the conversion factor is the dose (e.g., 100 mg/kg).

Let's assume we have a 20 kg (44 lb) animal and the dose of a drug for this species is 5 mg/kg. We can now determine the exact number of milligrams of drug to give this particular animal.

Proportion Method

$$\frac{X \text{ mg}}{20 \text{ kg}} = \frac{5 \text{ mg}}{\text{kg}}$$

$$X \text{ mg} \quad = 100 \text{ mg}$$

Cancel-Out Method

$$X \text{ mg} = 20 \cancel{\text{kg}} \times \frac{5 \text{ mg}}{\cancel{\text{kg}}}$$

$$X \text{ mg} \quad = 100 \text{ mg}$$

We now know that our 20 kg animal, given the drug at a dosage of 5 mg/kg, will receive 100 mg of the drug for a dose. The next step is to determine how much of the physical dose form (tablets, liquid) we must give to the animal in order to deliver 100 mg of drug.

DETERMINING HOW MANY UNITS OF THE DOSE FORM TO ADMINISTER

As described in Chapters 6 and 7, dose forms come with a certain "concentration" of drug within them. In the case of liquids, this concentration is usually expressed as a drug mass per volume of liquid medium (e.g., mg/mL, g/100 mL) or as a percentage solution (e.g., 2.27%, 15%). For solid dose forms it is the amount of drug within the solid unit (e.g., 50 mg/tablet, 100 mg/capsule, 6 mg/tsp of powder). The concentration of the drug becomes the conversion factor in determining how much of the physical dose form needs to be given.

The concentration conversion factor most used for liquid dose formulations is X mg per mL, although any unit of mass per volume can describe the concentration of drug in liquid. If the animal in our example above needs a liquid dose form, it can be administered either as an injectable or a liquid oral medication. The drug label, in this case, we will say, lists a concentration of 200 mg per mL (or think of it as 200 mg of drug *in* each mL of liquid). Therefore, we can set up the problem with the Unknown X expressed in milliliters (mL) of liquid, use the previously calculated drug dose of 100 mg as our known, and 200 mg/mL concentration of drug in liquid as the conversion factor.

Proportion Method

$$\frac{X \text{ mL}}{100 \text{ mg}} = \frac{1 \text{ mL}}{200 \text{ mg}}$$

$$X \text{ mL} = \frac{100 \text{ mg} \times 1 \text{ mL}}{200 \text{ mg}}$$

$$X \text{ mL} = \frac{1}{2} \text{ or } 0.5 \text{ mL}$$

Cancel-Out Method

$$X \text{ mL} = 100 \cancel{\text{ mg}} \times \frac{1 \text{ mL}}{200 \cancel{\text{ mg}}}$$

$$X \text{ mL} = 0.5 \text{ mL}$$

In order to use liquid dose form concentrations listed as *percentage solutions* (see Chapter 7), we have to perform an additional step in our calculations to change the percentage solution concentration to its equivalent concentration expressed as mg/mL. To do this requires remembering that X% solution is equivalent to X number of grams in 100 milliliters of fluid or that X% solution is equivalent to ten times X milligrams per milliliter.

$$X\% = \frac{X \text{ grams}}{100 \text{ mL}} = \frac{X \times 10 \text{ mg}}{\text{mL}}$$

Using these definitions, a 20% solution would then have 20 grams of drug per 100 mL of liquid, or 200 *milli*grams of drug per mL of liquid. Once we have converted a percentage solution into a mg/mL form, we can then use this concentration as the conversion factor in our calculation, as shown in the calculations above.

For tablets, the conversion factor most commonly used in calculations is X mg per tablet, although any mass of drug (grain, grams, etc.) per solid dose form unit (capsule, caplet, measured powder, etc.) can be used. If our 20 kg animal needs 100 mg of drug and the bottle containing the tablet lists the strength as 50 mg of drug per tablet, we can calculate how many tablets are needed. Our Unknown X is the number of tablets, the known value is dose of drug for this animal (100 mg), and the conversion factor is the concentration of the tablets (50 mg/tablet).

Proportion Method

$$\frac{X \text{ tablets}}{100 \text{ mg}} = \frac{1 \text{ tablet}}{50 \text{ mg}}$$

$$X \text{ tablets} = \frac{100 \text{ mg} \times 1 \text{ tablet}}{50 \text{ mg}}$$

$$X \text{ tablets} = 2 \text{ tablets}$$

Cancel-Out Method

$$X \text{ tablets} = 100 \text{ mg} \times \frac{1 \text{ tablet}}{50 \text{ mg}}$$

$$X \text{ tablets} = 2 \text{ tablets}$$

Notice that although the common way to verbally describe the tablet concentrations as 50 mg per tablet, in the calculation the conversion factor is set up so that it is 1 tablet per 50 mg. If we had written the conversion factor the other way, we would

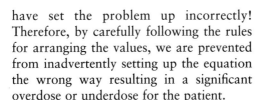
have set the problem up incorrectly! Therefore, by carefully following the rules for arranging the values, we are prevented from inadvertently setting up the equation the wrong way resulting in a significant overdose or underdose for the patient.

WHEN TABLET DOSES DON'T COME OUT EVEN

In the example problem above, the answer for the number of tablets needed was conveniently a whole number of tablets without any leftover fraction. In real life this seldom happens. If the animal weighed a few pounds more or less, the calculated number of tablets to be used per dose may have been 2.187 tablets or 1.745 tablets. It is difficult to imagine slicing off 0.187 of a tablet to be dispensed.

As a general rule of thumb, tablets should not be cut into anything less than 1/2. If your dose calculation requires 1/4 or 1/8 of a tablet, then either a different strength of tablet, if available, can be dispensed, or the required number of tablets can be rounded to the nearest 1/2 or whole tablet. Because many medications used in veterinary medicine are borrowed from the human side of medicine, the tablets are manufactured in strengths that are convenient for dosing a typical adult human. Because veterinary patients rarely weigh the same as a typical human adult and because doses in veterinary patients usually do not correlate with human doses, it is often necessary to adjust, or round, tablet sizes.

When rounding the calculated tablet dose to the nearest 1/2 or whole tablet, the following chart illustrates the appropriate rounding:

The fraction calculated tablet dose			The rounded tablet dose
up	to	1/2	1/2
1/2	to	3/4	1/2
3/4	to	1	1
1	to	1 1/4	1
1 1/4	to	1 1/2	1 1/2
1 1/2	to	1 3/4	1 1/2
1 3/4	to	2	2
etc.			etc.

DISPENSING MULTIPLE UNITS OF DRUG FORM

If a client is being dispensed medication to administer to an animal over several days, then we need to dispense multiple units of the dose form we just calculated. For example, if the animal was going to receive 2 tablets "q8h for 6 d," we have to decipher the drug order and determine the total amount to be dispensed. Although many times the total number of dose form units can be mentally calculated without writing the problem out, it is important to understand how to set up the problem using either the proportion method or the cancel-out method.

For calculating the total number of dose units to be dispensed, the Unknown X is going to be the X total tablets (or dose units) to be dispensed. The known value is the total number of doses to be used over the length of the dose regimen, and the conversion factor is the number of tablets (or dose units) per dose (in our example, 2 tablets per dose). The total number of doses (the known value in our equation) is determined by multiplying the number of doses per day by the number of days listed in the dosing orders. In our example, the dose orders stipulated "q8h for 6 d," which is "every 8 hours for six days." A "q8h" dose would be three doses per day.

$$\frac{\text{Number of Doses}}{1 \text{ Day}} \times \text{Number of Days}$$

$$\frac{3 \text{ Doses}}{\text{Day}} \times 6 \text{ Days}$$

18 TOTAL DOSES

Now that the total number of doses is determined, we use this value as the known value in either the proportional or cancel-out methods.

Proportion Method

$$\frac{\text{UNKNOWN UNIT}}{\text{KNOWN VALUE UNIT}} =$$

$$\frac{\text{CONVERSION FACTOR WITH SAME UNITS AS UNKNOWN}}{\text{CONVERSION FACTOR WITH SAME UNITS AS KNOWN}}$$

$$\frac{\text{X tablets}}{18 \text{ doses}} = \frac{2 \text{ tablets}}{\text{dose}}$$

$$\text{X tablets} = \frac{18 \text{ doses} \times 2 \text{ tablets}}{\text{dose}}$$

$$\text{X tablets} = \frac{18 \ \cancel{\text{doses}} \times 2 \text{ tablets}}{\cancel{\text{dose}}}$$

$$\text{X tablets} = 18 \times 2 \text{ tablets}$$

$$\text{X tablets} = 36 \text{ tablets}$$

Cancel-Out Method

$$\text{UNKNOWN UNIT} = \text{KNOWN VALUE} \times$$

$$\frac{\text{CONVERSION FACTOR WITH SAME UNITS AS UNKNOWN}}{\text{CONVERSION FACTOR WITH SAME UNITS AS KNOWN}}$$

$$\text{X tablets} = 18 \text{ doses} \times \frac{2 \text{ tablets}}{\text{dose}}$$

$$X \text{ tablets} = 18 \, \cancel{\text{doses}} \times \frac{2 \text{ tablets}}{\cancel{\text{dose}}}$$

$$X \text{ tablets} = 18 \times 2 \text{ tablets}$$

$$X \text{ tablets} = 36 \text{ tablets}$$

Again, to use the calculation for other dose form units, the same general procedures outlined above are used replacing tablets with the appropriate dose form unit.

THE MOST COMMON CALCULATION MISTAKE IN DISPENSING MULTIPLE UNITS

A student was given the following dose order for a 39 lb dog: "Give 5 mg/kg b.i.d. for 7 d." The medication comes in 50 mg tablets. The student went about filling the order in the following manner. Can you detect where the student went wrong in figuring out the total number of tablets to be dispensed?

STEP 1. The student first converted the dog's weight to kilograms.

$$X \text{ kg} = 39 \, \cancel{\text{lb}} \times \frac{1 \text{ kg}}{2.2 \, \cancel{\text{lb}}}$$

X kg = 17.72 kilograms, which was rounded to 17.7 kg

STEP 2. The dose was calculated for a 17.7 kg dog.

$$X \text{ mg drug} = 17.7 \cancel{\text{kg}} \times \frac{5 \text{ mg}}{\cancel{\text{kg}}}$$

$$X \text{ mg} = 88.5 \text{ mg}$$

STEP 3. The total number of doses was determined for "b.i.d. for 7 d."

$$\frac{2 \text{ doses}}{\text{day}} \times 7 \text{ days} = 14 \text{ total doses}$$

STEP 4. The student then figured the total dose for 14 doses.

$$X \text{ total mg} = 14 \text{ doses} \times \frac{88.5 \text{ mg}}{\text{dose}}$$

$$X \text{ total mg} = 14 \cancel{\text{doses}} \times \frac{88.5 \text{ mg}}{\cancel{\text{dose}}}$$

$$X \text{ total mg} = 14 \times 88.5 \text{ mg}$$

$$X \text{ total mg} = 1239 \text{ mg}$$

STEP 5. The student then calculated the total number of 50 mg tablets to be dispensed for this amount of drug (1239 milligrams).

$$X \text{ total tablets} = 1239 \text{ mg} \times \frac{1 \text{ tablet}}{50 \text{ mg}}$$

$$X \text{ total tablets} = 1239 \text{ mg} \times \frac{1 \text{ tablet}}{50 \text{ mg}}$$

$$X \text{ total tablets} = \frac{1239 \times 1 \text{ tablet}}{50}$$

$$X \text{ total tablets} = \frac{1239 \text{ tablet}}{50}$$

X total tablets = 24.78 tablets, which was rounded to 25 tablets

But wait! When the student went to figure out how many tablets the client was to give *per dose*, there was a problem! There were a total of 14 doses (b.i.d. for 7 d), thus a single dose would be 25 tablets divided by 14 doses.

25 tablets ÷ 14 = 1.7857142 tablet per dose

The math was all correct! So how did we end up with such an unusable tablet dose?

ANSWER: The student should have converted the 88.5 mg per dose to the number of tablets per dose after Step 2 of the calculations. Obviously if the milligrams of drug needed in the dose (88.5 mg) didn't exactly match the dose form (50 mg tablets) then some awkward fraction of tablet was going to be needed. When the student went on to calculate the total number of milligrams of drug, this fraction of tablet went into the calculation, resulting in a number at the end that was impractical to administer. Instead, the student should have rounded the 88.5 mg dose to the closest 1/2 or whole 50 mg tablet.

(for one dose)
$$\text{X tablet} = 88.5 \text{ mg} \times \frac{1 \text{ tablet}}{50 \text{ mg}}$$

(for one dose)
$$\text{X tablet} = 88.5 \, \cancel{\text{mg}} \times \frac{1 \text{ tablet}}{50 \, \cancel{\text{mg}}}$$

(for one dose)
$$\text{X tablet} = \frac{88.5 \times 1 \text{ tablet}}{50}$$

(for one dose)
$$\text{X tablet} = \frac{88.5 \text{ tablet}}{50}$$

(for one dose)
$$\text{X tablet} = 1.77 \text{ tablet}$$

1.77 tablet is closer to 2.0 tablets than it is to 1.5 tablets, so the number of tablets given *per dose* is going to be 2 tablets. There are 14 doses total to be given over the 7 days, so the total number of tablets to be dispensed would be:

(whole regimen)

$$\text{X tablets} = 14 \text{ doses} \times \frac{2 \text{ tablet}}{\text{dose}}$$

(whole regimen)

X tablets = 14 × 2 tablets

(whole regimen)

X tablets = 28 tablets

Remember: whenever calculating a total number of dose units to be dispensed over the span of a dosage regimen, always convert the *amount of drug per dose* into the *number of dose units per dose* before determining the total dose units to be dispensed!

SECTION I

PRACTICE PROBLEMS

(Answers are at the end of the chapter.)

1) Convert the animal's weight to the appropriate units:

    a) 30 kg   =   _____ lb

    b) 88 lb   =   _____ kg

    c) 1348 lb   =   _____ kg

    d) 0.0321 kg =   _____ g

    e) 0.032 lb   =   _____ g

2) Determine how much drug (in mg) each animal needs:

   a) 43 lb dog, dose is 2 mg/lb =
     _____ mg

   b) 11 lb cat, dose is 5 mg/kg =
     _____ mg

   c) 896 lb horse, dose is 2 mg/kg =
     _____ mg

   d) 0.5 kg rat, dose is 0.25 mg/kg =
     _____ mg

3) Determine how many tablets per dose each animal needs. Each tablet may be broken into nothing smaller than 1/2 tablet.

   a) 67 lb dog, dose is 10 mg/kg, 200 mg tablet = _____ tablets per dose

   b) 8 lb cat, dose is 5 mg/kg, 10 mg tablet = _____ tablets per dose

   c) 950 lb horse, dose is 1 mg/kg, 200 mg tablet = _____ tablets per dose

   d) 1 kg guinea pig, dose is 10 mg/lb, 20 mg tablet = _____ tablets per dose

4) Determine what volume of liquid per dose each animal needs. Round to nearest 1/10 mL:

a) 48 lb dog, dose is 25 mg/kg, bottle
   concentration 250 mg/mL =
   _____ mL

b) 6 lb cat, dose is 20 mg/kg, bottle
   concentration 30 mg/mL =
   _____ mL

c) 1000 lb horse, dose is 1 mg/kg, bottle
   concentration 100 mg/mL =
   _____ mL

d) 3 lb rabbit, dose is 10 mg/kg, bottle
   concentration is 15 mg/mL =
   _____ mL

5) Determine what volume of liquid per
dose each animal needs given the percentage solution of the drug. Round to the
nearest 1/10 mL:

a) 22 lb dog, 25 mg/kg, 25% solution =
   _____ mL per dose

b) 765 lb heifer, 10 mg/kg, 50%
   solution = _____ mL per dose

6) Determine the total number of tablets
dispensed. Tablets can be broken into nothing smaller than 1/2 tablet:

a) 110 lb dog, dose 5 mg/kg q8h 10d
   PO, 250 mg tablets =
   _____ tablets

    b) 10.5 lb cat, dose 50 mg/kg b.i.d. 5d
       PO, 100 mg tablets =
       _____ tablets

SECTION II DOSING WITH THE HYPODERMIC SYRINGE

Liquid dose forms can be administered orally or by injection. In either situation, the liquid dose form is most often loaded into a syringe for administration. In order for the correct amount of drug to be delivered, the proper dose calculation must be performed, and the amount of drug pulled into the syringe must equal the volume calculated. Reading the syringe properly helps ensure that the proper volume of medication will be administered.

TYPES OF SYRINGES USED IN VETERINARY MEDICINE

Plastic syringes used in veterinary medicine range in total capacity from small 1 cc (1 mL) syringes, sometimes called tuberculin syringes, all the way up to 60 cc syringes. Another type of dosing syringe often used in livestock production facilities is the multidose syringe or "dose gun," which is capable of delivering measured amounts of medication repeatedly with each squeeze of the spring-loaded trigger. Large metallic dosing syringes with blunted metal tips are also used with horses and livestock to administer liquid oral medications.

One special type of syringe, the insulin syringe, is sometimes used in veterinary medicine. The insulin syringe is special in that the markings on the syringe barrel are not in standard metric volumetric units, but instead are designed to measure units of insulin that correspond to a particular standardized concentration of insulin. Multidose vials of insulin typically come in standardized concentrations of 40 units per mL or 100 units per mL. A "unit" is based on the activity of the insulin. Therefore, the abbreviation U-100 on either a syringe or vial of insulin refers to the standard concentration of 100 units (U) of insulin per mL (cc). A U-100 vial of insulin requires a U-100 syringe for accurate administration, and U-40 insulin requires a U-40 insulin syringe. Because each insulin syringe has a volume capacity of 1 mL, the markings on the U-40 syringe range from 0 to 40, and the markings on the U-100 syringe range from 0 to 100.

SYRINGE UNITS OF MEASUREMENT

Figure 8.1 illustrates the markings on a standard 3 cc (3 mL) syringe. The markings show increments of 0.1 (one-tenth) of a cc. Most larger syringes, like the 35 cc syringe shown in Figure 8.2, have increments of 1 cc or 1 mL. Although a dose of 2.3 mL would be quite easy to accurately draw into a 3 cc syringe, the same amount might be off by a 1/2 of a mL or more if drawn into the 35 cc syringe. Therefore, it is important to choose a syringe that allows whatever degree of accuracy is needed by the dosing orders.

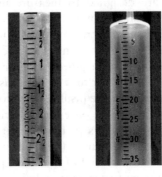

Figure 8.1 3 cc syringe   Figure 8.2 35 cc syringe

Notice the markings on the 20 mL (Figure 8.3) and 60 cc (Figure 8.4) syringes.

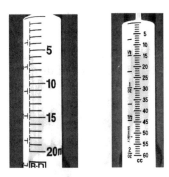

Figure 8.3 20 mL syringe   Figure 8.4 60 cc syringe

In both of these syringes there are an additional set of marks and numbers to the left of the incremental scale for cubic centimeters or milliliters. It is not unusual to find two scales of increments on a syringe to facilitate dosing a drug. For these two particular syringes, the alternate scale is in fluid ounces (oz). The fluid ounce marks on the 60 cc syringe are in 1/4 ounce increments, and the marks on the 20 mL syringe are in 1/8 fluid ounce increments. Sometimes the 3cc syringes will contain a scale that is labeled with a modified *M* character to indicate the units on the scale. This scale is in "minims" and is represented by the symbol ♏. A minim is an old apothecary system measurement and is approximately equal to 1 drop. The scale is rarely used in veterinary medicine, and for the purposes of this textbook will not be considered.

MEASURING THE AMOUNT OF LIQUID IN A SYRINGE

Figure 8.5 shows a 3 cc syringe partially filled with 2.7 mL or cc of drug.

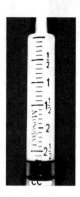

Figure 8.5 3 cc syringe partially filled with 2.7 mL of drug

When withdrawing the drug from the vial into the syringe, the volume of drug in the syringe is always read by the edge of the black plunger closest to the syringe hub (the hub is where the needle attaches). Notice that the rubber plunger has more than one ring of rubber to provide an airtight seal. Sometimes beginning students may confuse the ring closest to the plunger for the indicator at which they are to measure the drug volume.

It is important to remember that if air

bubbles become mixed with the drug in the syringe barrel, the amount of drug actually in the syringe cannot be accurately measured. In those situations it is necessary to tap the barrel of the syringe several times, usually with a flick of the finger against the barrel, while the syringe is being held with the hub end up. This will usually allow the air bubble(s) to rise to the hub where the air can be expelled with the minimum of drug lost.

When injecting the drug into the animal, make sure the plunger of the syringe goes as far forward to the hub as possible. Note that some small amount of drug will always remain in the hub itself even after the plunger has been fully pressed into the barrel of the syringe. This is of no consequence to the amount of drug administered, because the markings on the syringe barrel account for the amount of drug lost in this "dead space" in the hub of the syringe. Do remember, however, that for potentially dangerous drugs (like antineoplastic, cancer-fighting drugs) some of this drug will remain in the syringe and the chance for accidental exposure to the drug by the veterinary professional is possible.

SECTION II
PRACTICE PROBLEMS
(Answers are at the end of the chapter.)

1. For each of these syringes, indicate the volume of medication the syringe contains.

a)

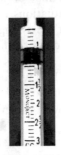

b)

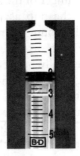

c)

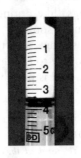

2. For each of these syringes, indicate the volume of medication the syringe contains.

a)

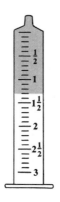

b)

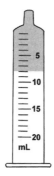

c)

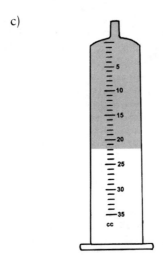

3. For each of these syringes below, make a mark on the picture that indicates where the volume of drug would be.

a)

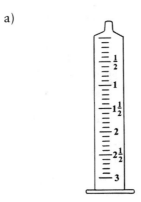

2.5 cc

b)

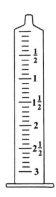

0.8 mL

c)

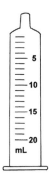

18 cc

d)

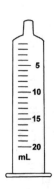

3 mL

e)

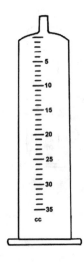

14 cc

f)

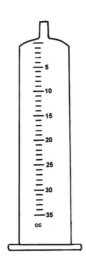

31 mL

ANSWERS FOR PRACTICE PROBLEMS

SECTION I

1) a) 66 lb   d) 32.1 g

   b) 40 kg   e) 14.5 g

   c) 612.73 kg

2) a) 86 mg   c) 814.5 mg

   b) 25 mg   d) 0.125 mg

3) a)

$$67 \text{ lb} \times \frac{\text{kg}}{2.2 \text{ lb}} \times \frac{10 \text{ mg}}{\text{kg}} \times \frac{1 \text{ tablet}}{200 \text{ mg}} =$$

1.523 tablets = 1.5 tablets

b)

$$8 \text{ lb} \times \frac{\text{kg}}{2.2 \text{ lb}} \times \frac{5 \text{ mg}}{\text{kg}} \times \frac{1 \text{ tablet}}{10 \text{ mg}} =$$

1.82 tablets = 2 tablets

c)

$$950 \text{ lb} \times \frac{\text{kg}}{2.2 \text{ lb}} \times \frac{1 \text{ mg}}{\text{kg}} \times \frac{1 \text{ tablet}}{200 \text{ mg}} =$$

2.16 tablets = 2 tablets

d)

$$1 \text{ kg} \times \frac{2.2 \text{ lb}}{\text{kg}} \times \frac{10 \text{ mg}}{\text{lb}} \times \frac{1 \text{ tablet}}{20 \text{ mg}} =$$

1.1 tablet = 1 tablet

4) a)

$$48 \text{ lb} \times \frac{\text{kg}}{2.2 \text{ lb}} \times \frac{25 \text{mg}}{\text{kg}} \times \frac{1 \text{ mL}}{250 \text{ mg}} =$$

2.2 mL

b)

$$6 \text{ lb} \times \frac{\text{kg}}{2.2 \text{ lb}} \times \frac{20 \text{ mg}}{\text{kg}} \times \frac{1 \text{ mL}}{30 \text{ mg}} =$$

1.8 mL

c)

$$1000 \text{ lb} \times \frac{\text{kg}}{2.2 \text{ lb}} \times \frac{1 \text{ mg}}{\text{kg}} \times \frac{1 \text{ mL}}{100 \text{ mg}} =$$

4.5 mL

d)

$$3 \text{ lb} \times \frac{\text{kg}}{2.2 \text{ lb}} \times \frac{10 \text{ mg}}{\text{kg}} \times \frac{1 \text{ mL}}{15 \text{ mg}} =$$

0.9 mL

5) a)

$$22 \text{ lb} \times \frac{\text{kg}}{2.2 \text{ lb}} \times \frac{25 \text{ mg}}{\text{kg}} \times \frac{1 \text{ mL}}{250 \text{ mg}} =$$

1.0 mL (25% = 250 mg/mL)

$$22 \text{ lb} \times$$

$$\frac{\text{kg}}{2.2 \text{ lb}} \times \frac{25 \text{ mg}}{\text{kg}} \times \frac{1 \text{ g}}{1000 \text{ mg}} \times \frac{100 \text{ mL}}{25 \text{ g}} =$$

1.0 mL (25g/100 mL)

b)

$$765 \text{ lb} \times \frac{\text{kg}}{2.2 \text{ lb}} \times \frac{10 \text{ mg}}{\text{kg}} \times \frac{1 \text{ mL}}{500 \text{ mg}} =$$

6.95 mL = 7.0 mL (50% = 500 mg/mL)

6) a)

$$110 \text{ lb} \times \frac{\text{kg}}{2.2 \text{ lb}} \times \frac{5 \text{ mg}}{\text{kg}} \times \frac{1 \text{ tablet}}{250 \text{ mg}} =$$

1.0 tablet per dose

$$\frac{1 \text{ tablet}}{\text{dose}} \times \frac{3 \text{ doses}}{\text{day}} \times 10 \text{ days} =$$

30 tablets total

b)

$$10.5 \text{ lb} \times \frac{\text{kg}}{2.2 \text{ lb}} \times \frac{50 \text{ mg}}{\text{kg}} \times \frac{1 \text{ tablet}}{100 \text{ mg}} =$$

2.38 tablets = 2.5 tablets per dose

$$\frac{2.5 \text{ tablets}}{\text{dose}} \times \frac{2 \text{ doses}}{\text{day}} \times 5 \text{ days} =$$

25 tablets total

SECTION II

1) a)   0.5 cc

   b)   2 cc

   c)   3.4 cc

2) a) 1.3 cc

   b) 8 cc

   c) 22 cc

3) a)

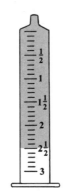

   b)

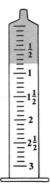

c)

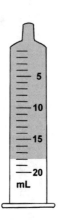

d)

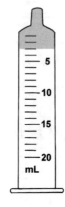

e)

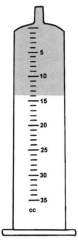

f)

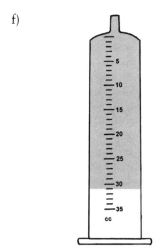

CHAPTER 8 PROBLEMS

1) Convert the animal's weight to the appropriate units:

    a) 23.3 kg = _____ lb

    b) 1088 lb = _____ kg

    c) 34 lb = _____ kg

    d) 3092 g = _____ kg

    e) 0.08732 lb = _____ g

2) Determine how much drug (in mg) each animal needs.

a) 65 lb dog, dose is 3 mg/lb
    = _____ mg

    b) 8.5 lb cat, dose is 50 mg/kg
       = _____ mg

    c) 923 lb horse, dose is 0.5 mg/kg
       = _____ mg

    d) 0.75 kg guinea pig, dose is 0.35 mg/kg
       = _____ mg

3) Determine how many tablets per dose each animal needs. Each tablet may be broken into pieces no smaller than 1/2 tablet.

a) 33.5 lb dog, dose is 20 mg/kg, 200 mg
   tablet = _____ tablets per dose

b) 6.25 lb cat, dose is 15 mg/kg, 20 mg
   tablet = _____ tablets per dose

c) 849 lb horse, dose is 25 mg/kg, 5 gram
   tablet = _____ tablets per dose

d) 0.66 kg rat, dose is 3.25 mg/lb, 2.0 mg
   tablet = _____ tablets per dose

4) Determine what volume of liquid per
dose each animal needs. Round to nearest
1/10 mL.

a) 24 lb dog, dose is 25 mg/kg, bottle
   concentration 125 mg/mL
   = _____ mL

b) 9.75 lb cat, dose is 20 mg/kg, bottle
   concentration 250 mg/mL
   = _____ mL

c) 982 lb horse, dose is 10 mg/kg, bottle
   concentration 1.5 g/mL
   = _____ mL

d) 2.8 lb rabbit, dose is 150 mg/kg, bottle concentration is 125 mg/mL
   = _____ mL

5) Determine what volume of liquid per dose each animal needs given the percentage solution of the drug. Round to the nearest 1/10 mL.

a) 36 lb dog, 20 mg/kg, 20% solution
= _____mL per dose

b) 265 lb sow, 7.50 mg/kg, 42.5%
solution = _____ mL per dose

6) Determine the total number of tablets dispensed. Tablets can be broken into nothing smaller than 1/2 tablet.

a) 86.5 lb dog, dose 15 mg/kg q6h 12d PO,
200 mg tablets = _____ tablets

b) 9 lb cat, dose 50 mg/kg b.i.d. 5d PO, 100
mg tablets = _____ tablets

c) 600 lb cow, 10 mg/kg s.i.d. 10d PO, 3
gram tablets = _____ tablets

d) 1090 lb stallion, 1.5 mg/kg q12h 7d,
400 mg tablets = _____ tablets

e) 12.4 kg dog, 6.8 mg/lb t.i.d. 15d, 75 mg
tablets = _____ tablets

f) 47 lb dog, 2 mg/kg s.i.d. 180d, 1/2 grain
tablets = _____ tablets

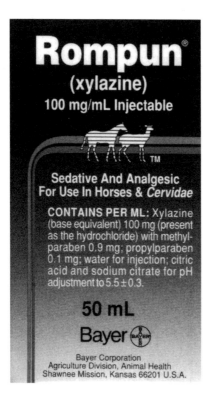

Rompun®
(xylazine)
100 mg/mL Injectable

TM

Sedative And Analgesic
For Use In Horses & Cervidae

CONTAINS PER ML: Xylazine
(base equivalent) 100 mg (present
as the hydrochloride) with methyl-
paraben 0.9 mg; propylparaben
0.1 mg; water for injection; citric
acid and sodium citrate for pH
adjustment to 5.5 ± 0.3.

50 mL
Bayer ⊛

Bayer Corporation
Agriculture Division, Animal Health
Shawnee Mission, Kansas 66201 U.S.A.

7) The veterinarian needs to use the sedative analgesic drug above on a 900 pound
horse and a 900 pound bull. The dose for
the horse is 1.1 mg/kg IV and for the bull it
is 0.05 mg/kg IV. Determine the number of
milliliters of this drug that will need to be
given to the equine and the bovine patient.
List the size of syringes you would use for
each patient.

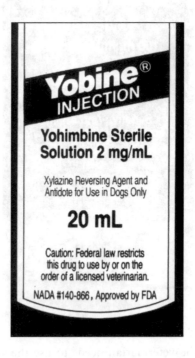

8) Once in awhile a bovine patient receives an equine equivalent dose of xylazine shown in the previous problem. Such a high dose would produce significant toxic signs in the bovine patient. To reverse the effect, yohimbine is given at a dose of 0.125 mg/kg IV. How many cubic centimeters of yohimbine would the 900 bull in problem 7 need?

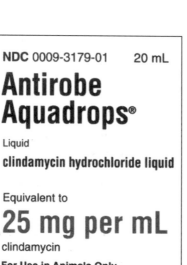

NDC 0009-3179-01   20 mL

Antirobe Aquadrops®

Liquid

clindamycin hydrochloride liquid

Equivalent to

25 mg per mL

clindamycin

For Use in Animals Only

Caution: Federal (USA) law
restricts this drug to use by or on
the order of a licensed veterinarian.
NADA #135-940, Approved by FDA

Upjohn

9) You have a dog and cat needing to be treated with this antibiotic for a deep wound and an abscess respectively. The dog, "Max," weighs 23 pounds, while "Felinsha," the cat, weighs 8 1/2 pounds. The dose for Max is 6.5 mg/kg q12h PO for 5 days, while the dose for Felinsha is 10 mg/kg q12h PO for 8 days.

a) What is the single dose (in milliliters) for both Max and Felinsha?

b) How many milliliters total would each pet need to complete the prescribed dose regimen?

c) How many boxes of Antirobe would Max need to finish his dose regimen?

d) How many boxes would Felinsha need?

10) "Pepe" the Chihuahua has a skin infection that needs to be treated with Cefa-Drops®. "Jocko," the terrier-mix that lives with Pepe, has a similar infection and will be treated with the same drug. The kitten, "Boris," who actually runs the house and bosses both of the dogs, has a similar infection on his face. The canine dose is 22 mg/kg b.i.d. PO. The feline dose is 22 mg/kg q8h PO. Boris weighs 5.5 pounds, Pepe weighs 9 pounds, and Jocko is the relative heavyweight at 29 pounds. Boris needs to be on this drug for 7 days, and the dogs need to be on the medication for 10 days.

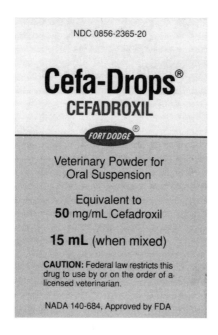

NDC 0856-2365-20

Cefa-Drops®
CEFADROXIL

FORT DODGE®

Veterinary Powder for
Oral Suspension

Equivalent to
50 mg/mL Cefadroxil

15 mL (when mixed)

CAUTION: Federal law restricts this
drug to use by or on the order of a
licensed veterinarian.

NADA 140-684, Approved by FDA

a) What are the individual animal doses in milliliters?

b) How much total milliliters of this drug would need to be dispensed to treat all three animals for their prescribed time?

c) How many boxes of this formulation of drug would need to be dispensed to cover the medication needed for all the dose regimens?

d) If each box of medication sold for $7.50 each, what would be the cost to the owners of these pets?

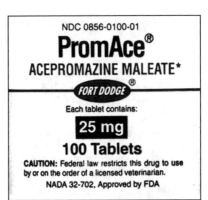

11) Mrs. Jones is going to be traveling with her three dogs and one cat. She wants to get some acepromazine tranquilizer for all the animals. The acepromazine tablets above are difficult to split into halves, so this dose form is going to have to be dispensed as full tablets. Mrs. Jones's dogs weigh 30 pounds, 45 pounds, and 85 pounds. The cat weighs 8 pounds. The canine dose for this drug is a dose range of 0.55 to 2.2 mg/kg PO PRN. The cat dose is 1.1 to 2.2 mg/kg. All doses should fit within the specified dose range, and the tablet size used is the one indicated on the bottle.

a) What would be the minimum dose (in milligrams) for each dog based on the lower end of the dose range?

b) What would be the maximum dose (in milligrams) for each dog based on the upper end of the dose range?

c) How many full tablets should each of the three dogs be dispensed for tranquilization?
d) If the tablets sell for $0.75 each, plus a dispensing fee of $3.00 per animal, what would be the total cost to Mrs. Jones for the three dogs?
e) What is the range of doses (in milligrams) for the cat?
f) Should this dose form (25 mg tablets) be used in the cat?

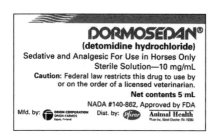

12) The veterinarian wants to sedate an 850 pound horse and a 375 pony. The dose for this drug in horses and ponies is 20 to 40 micrograms per kilogram. The lower dose will provide sedation for 30 to 90 minutes, and the higher dose will provide sedation for 90 to 120 minutes.

a) 20 to 40 micrograms/kilogram (mcg/kg) is equivalent to how many mg/kg?

b) What dose, in milliliters, would the horse and pony each need to provide 30 minutes of sedation?

c) What dose, in milliliters, would each animal need for up to 2 hours of sedation?

d) Would one bottle be sufficient volume to provide sedation for up to 2 hours for both animals?

CALCULATING INTRAVENOUS INFUSIONS

Objectives
The student will be able to do the following:

1. Determine the flow rate for an infusion by observing the drip rate in the drip chamber.
2. Determine the volume of fluid that will be infused given an infusion rate.
3. Determine what infusion rate (drip rate) is needed in order to deliver a set volume of fluid within a prescribed period of time.
3. Determine the stop time for IV infusions based on volume or dose of medication to be administered.

Drugs and intravenous fluids are sometimes administered over a period of time in order to ensure that the medication achieves and sustains therapeutic concentrations while avoiding unnecessarily high peak concentrations and their subsequent toxic reactions or side effects. Therefore, the veterinary professional needs to understand how to calculate infusion rates for medications and fluids administered intravenously over time.

SECTION I INTRAVENOUS INFUSION OF MEDICATION

Drug orders may prescribe administering an intravenous drug either by infusion (drug dripped into the patient over time) or a bolus (drug administered quickly in a push). Drug orders prescribing IV infusion describe the amount of drug to be administered and the route of administration, plus a time factor for administration. For example:

35 mg given intravenously over 5 minutes

250 mL of the 10mg/mL concentration administered IV over 2 hours

In order to administer the drug within the designated period of time, the medication must flow into the patient at a particular rate. The veterinary professional must be able to interpret the observed flow rate, translate that observation into a volume delivered per unit of time, and then be able to adjust the rate to meet the prescribed time frame for the intravenous infusion.

TYPES OF IV ADMINISTRATION SETS

Several types of IV administration sets are used in veterinary medicine; see Figure 9.1.

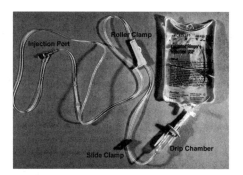

Figure 9.1 Intravenous administration set

At one end of the intravenous tubing is some means of attaching or inserting the IV administration set into an intravenous fluid bag or bottle. Just below the point where the IV tubing attaches to the fluid bag or bottle is a clear plastic chamber called the *drip chamber* through which the drops of fluid or drug can be observed passing from the fluid bag/bottle into the IV tubing.

The intravenous tubing itself usually has either (or both) a *roller clamp* or *slide clamp* to regulate the flow of fluid through the IV tubing. An *injection port* may also be incorporated into the IV tubing for injecting drugs into the flowing IV fluids. The injection port most commonly consists of a Y-shaped plastic tube with a rubber stopper on one of the branches of the Y through which medication can be injected. At the terminus of the IV tubing is the hub that inserts into a needle or catheter.

To start the fluid flowing through the IV line, the slide clamp is moved or the wheel on the roller clamp rolled. Once the clamp is opened, drops can be observed dropping from the fluid bag/bottle into the liquid in the drip chamber.

To be able to observe the IV fluid dripping from the bag/bottle through the drip chamber (and thus be able to calculate the rate of flow for the IV fluids), the drip chamber must be only half filled with fluid. Filling the chamber all the way prevents observation of the drips dropping through the chamber, and not filling the chamber may allow air in the chamber to flow along with the IV fluids into the patient. To fill the drip chamber after attaching the IV tubing to the fluid bag or bottle, hang the bag/bottle from an IV stand with the drip chamber below the bag/bottle, squeeze the drip chamber slightly to expel some of the air from the drip chamber into the IV bag or bottle, then release the drip chamber. The drip chamber will partially fill with liquid.

DETERMINING THE VOLUME OF FLUID DELIVERED

To determine the volume of fluid being delivered through an IV administration set, we need to know the following:

1. The rate of drips dropping through the drip chamber (drips per unit of time)
2. The calibration of the IV administration set (drips per milliliter)

To determine the volume of fluid passing through the IV line, the number of drops observed in the drip chamber needs to be converted into milliliters. Each IV administration set is calibrated so that a set number of drips observed passing through the drip chamber equals one milliliter (1 mL) of fluid delivered. The conversion is usually listed on the package material that contains the IV administration set.

The most common forms of the standard, or *macrodrip*, IV administration sets are calibrated so that 15 or 20 drops equal one milliliter. There are also some macrodrip IV administration sets that deliver 10 drops as one milliliter. The microdrip IV sets (sometimes referred to as pediatric drip sets) are usually calibrated as 60 drops equals one milliliter. Remember that "gtt" is the abbreviation for drops, or drips, used in prescriptions and drug orders; therefore the calibration listed on the package may appear as "20 gtt/mL" or "60 gtt/mL."

Let's illustrate how a flow rate for an IV administration set can be determined. Say we are using a standard or macrodrip IV administration set that is calibrated so that 20 drops seen in the drip chamber equals 1 milliliter (20 gtt/mL). Let us say further that we observed 40 drips passing through the drip chamber each minute. We now need to identify how many milliliters of fluid were dripped into the patient during one minute.

To set up a this problem using the cancel-out method, we set the Unknown X (what we want to find out) to be the number of milliliters of IV fluid passed in one minute. The known value would be the observed drips in the drip chamber in one minute, and the conversion factor is the drips/mL (gtt/mL) calibration of the IV administration set.

UNKNOWN = KNOWN VALUE × CONVERSION FACTOR

X mL = drips (gtt) × IV set calibration (mL/gtt)

$$X \text{ mL} = 40 \text{ drips (gtt)} \times \frac{1 \text{ ml}}{20 \text{ gtt}}$$

Notice how the equation is set up so that the units of gtt in the numerator would be cancelled out by the gtt in the denominator, leaving only the units of milliliters (which is the unit of measurement for the answer in this problem).

$$X \text{ mL} = 40 \; \cancel{\text{drips (gtt)}} \times \frac{1 \text{ mL}}{20 \; \cancel{\text{gtt}}}$$

$$X \text{ mL} = 40 \ \times \frac{1 \text{ mL}}{20}$$

$$X \text{ mL} = \frac{40 \text{ mL}}{20}$$

$$X \text{ mL} = 2 \text{ mL}$$

Therefore, 2 milliliters would have passed through the drip chamber and into the patient in one minute. The 2 milliliter answer was actually 2 milliliters *per minute,* and the 40 drips observed in the drip chamber were actually 40 drips *per minute.* To reflect the time involved in the passage of the drips and milliliters, we could have set up the equation to include the time unit of one minute, as shown below.

$$X \text{ mL} = 40 \text{ drips (gtt)} \ \times \frac{1 \text{mL}}{20 \text{gtt}}$$

is equivalent to

$$\frac{X \text{mL}}{\text{minute}} = \frac{40 \text{ drips (gtt)}}{\text{minute}} \times \frac{1 \text{ mL}}{20 \text{ gtt}}$$

We can incorporate units of time in our equations to calculate the milliliter flow rate (mL/unit of time) after observing the number of drips passing in a variety of time frames such as 10 seconds, 3 minutes, or

0.25 hour. To perform the calculation using the standard format for the cancel-out method, we set our Unknown X to be X milliliters *per unit of time* (e.g., 30 seconds, 2 hour, 15 minutes, etc.), set the known value to be the number of drips observed *per unit of time*, and set the conversion factor to be calibration of the IV set in *milliliters per drip*.

For example, if we observed 30 drips passing through the drip chamber in 10 seconds for an IV set that was calibrated to 15 gtt/mL, we set up the calculation as follows:

UNKNOWN = KNOWN VALUE × CONVERSION FACTOR

$$\frac{X \text{ mL}}{\text{unit of time}} =$$

$$\frac{\text{drips (gtt)}}{\text{unit of time}} \times \text{IV set calibration} \left(\frac{\text{mL}}{\text{gtt}}\right)$$

$$\frac{X \text{ mL}}{10 \text{ seconds}} = \frac{30 \text{ drips}}{10 \text{ seconds}} \times \frac{1 \text{ mL}}{15 \text{ drips}}$$

$$\frac{X \text{ mL}}{10 \text{ seconds}} = \frac{30 \; \cancel{\text{drips}}}{10 \text{ seconds}} \times \frac{1 \text{ mL}}{15 \; \cancel{\text{drips}}}$$

$$\frac{X \text{ mL}}{10 \text{ seconds}} = \frac{30 \times 1 \text{ mL}}{10 \text{ seconds} \times 15}$$

$$\frac{X \text{ mL}}{10 \text{ seconds}} = \frac{30 \text{ mL}}{10 \text{ seconds} \times 15}$$

$$\frac{X \text{ mL}}{10 \text{ seconds}} = \frac{2 \text{ mL}}{10 \text{ seconds}}$$

Just as in all of the previous example problems, the units on the left side of the equation (mL/10 seconds) must be the same as the units on the right side of the equation. If in the third or fourth step above, the student would have multiplied the "10 seconds × 15" together to get 150 seconds, the numerators on either side of the equation would not have been the same.

$$\frac{X \text{ mL}}{10 \text{ seconds}} = \frac{30 \text{ mL}}{10 \text{ seconds} \times 15}$$

$$\frac{X \text{ mL}}{10 \text{ seconds}} = \frac{30 \text{ mL}}{150 \text{ seconds}}$$

$$\frac{X \text{ mL}}{10 \text{ seconds}} = \frac{0.2 \text{ mL}}{1 \text{ second}}$$

The answer on the right side of the equation tells us how many milliliters are flowing per second. However, the left side of the equation is asking how many milliliters are flowing into the patient in *10 seconds*. Therefore, to determine the flow rate for 10 seconds (and to make the denominators on both sides of the equation agree with each other), we have to multiply the right side of the equation by 10/10.

$$\frac{X \text{ mL}}{10 \text{ seconds}} = \frac{0.2 \text{ mL}}{1 \text{ second}} \times \frac{10}{10}$$

$$\frac{X \text{ mL}}{10 \text{ seconds}} = \frac{2 \text{ mL}}{10 \text{ seconds}}$$

The flow rate of 0.2 mL/second is exactly the same value as the flow rate of 2 mL/10 seconds! Mathematically we know this is true because we converted the 0.2 mL/second to 2 mL/10 seconds by multiplying the numerator and denominator of 0.2 mL/second by 10/10. We know 10/10 has a value of 1 (see earlier chapters on fractions and reciprocals if you have questions about this) because any number multiplied by one equals itself; so 0.2 mL/second = 2 mL/10 seconds.

Note that a more accurate assessment of flow rate through the IV line can be made by observing the number of drips passing through the drip chamber over a longer period of time. For example, calculating the flow rate based on the number of drips passing through the chamber in 30 seconds will provide a more accurate assessment of the fluid flow rate than counting drips for 5 seconds. The reason for this is that the number of drips observed in 5 seconds rarely ends as a "whole" drip. Instead, 1/4, 1/2, 3/4, or any fraction worth of drips may have "flowed" from the bottle into the drip chamber, but because we don't see a fraction of a drip fall through the chamber, any fractional drip is discarded in the calculation. A 1/2 drip error every 5 seconds would expand to a 6 drips per minute error, whereas a 1/2 drip error every 30 seconds results in only an error of 1 drip per minute.

CONVERTING FLOW RATE BETWEEN TIME UNITS

It is important for the veterinary professional to be able to accurately convert from drips per second to the equivalent drips per minute or to convert milliliters per minute to the equivalent milliliters per hour so that IV fluid flow rates can be properly set, monitored, and adjusted.

To convert a given drips or milliliters per time unit to its equivalent value in another time unit (e.g., convert drips per 15 seconds to drips per minute), make the given rate the known value, the new rate the Unknown X, and the time-to-time conversion (minutes to seconds, minutes to hours) the conversion factor in the equation. For example, if we have observed that a given flow rate is 1.5 milliliters in 15 seconds and we want to know what the equivalent milliliter flow rate would be in 1 minute, we would set up the equation as follows:

$$\text{UNKNOWN} = \text{KNOWN VALUE} \times \text{CONVERSION FACTOR}$$

Rate to Be = Rate Given × Time Unit Conversion
Determined (mL/Time Unit 2) (Time Unit 2/Time Unit 1)
(mL/Time Unit 1)

$$\frac{\text{X mL}}{1\ \text{minute}} = \frac{1.5\ \text{mL}}{15\ \text{seconds}} \times \frac{60\ \text{seconds}}{1\ \text{minute}}$$

$$\frac{\text{X mL}}{1\ \text{minute}} = \frac{1.5\ \text{mL}}{15\ \cancel{\text{seconds}}} \times \frac{60\ \cancel{\text{seconds}}}{1\ \text{minute}}$$

$$\frac{\text{X mL}}{1\ \text{minute}} = \frac{1.5\ \text{mL} \times 60}{15 \times 1\ \text{minute}}$$

$$\frac{\text{X mL}}{1\ \text{minute}} = \frac{90\ \text{mL}}{15\ \text{minutes}}$$

$$\frac{\text{X mL}}{1\ \text{minute}} = \frac{6\ \text{mL}}{1\ \text{minute}}$$

The units in the denominators on each side of the equation are the same, so our calculation doesn't need to be adjusted further. Therefore, a flow rate of 1.5 mL every 15 seconds is equivalent to 6 mL per minute. A similar format can be used to convert minutes to hours, hours to seconds, and so forth.

DETERMINING THE TOTAL VOLUME
DELIVERED OVER TIME

Given a particular drip rate, we should be able to calculate what volume of IV fluids or drug will be delivered by a set period of time. For example, if we had determined that the flow rate through an IV line was set at 15 mL per minute, we can determine how much volume will be delivered at that rate in 30 minutes, 1 hour, or 8 hours by using the 15 mL/minute as the known, the X mL/30 minutes as the Unknown, and the relationship between our two units of time as our conversion factor. Let's demonstrate how to set up to calculate the volume delivered at 30 minutes, 1 hour, and 8 hours, given the rate of 15 mL/minute.

Volume delivered in 30 minutes at a rate of 15 mL/minute:

$$\frac{X \text{ mL}}{30 \text{ minutes}} = \frac{15 \text{ mL}}{\text{minute}} \times \frac{1 \text{ minute}}{1 \text{ minute}}$$

In this example, there isn't a need to convert to a different time unit. Both of the answers are in minutes. So the 1 minute/1 minute component could be eliminated because its numerical value is 1.

$$\frac{X \text{ mL}}{30 \text{ minutes}} = \frac{15 \text{ mL}}{\text{minute}}$$

We do see that the denominators on either side of the equation are not the same. To correct this, we need to multiply the right side by 30/30 so that both sides of the equation will have *30 minutes* in the denominator.

$$\frac{X \text{ mL}}{30 \text{ minutes}} = \frac{15 \text{ mL}}{\text{minute}} \times \frac{30}{30}$$

$$\frac{X \text{ mL}}{30 \text{ minutes}} = \frac{450 \text{ mL}}{30 \text{ minutes}}$$

Therefore, at the rate of 15 mL/minute, in 30 minutes 450 milliliters of fluid will have been delivered.

Volume delivered in 1 hour at a rate of 15 mL/minute:

$$\frac{X \text{ mL}}{1 \text{ hour}} = \frac{15 \text{ mL}}{\text{minute}} \times \frac{60 \text{ minutes}}{1 \text{ hour}}$$

In this case the time unit on the left side of the equation (hours) is different than the time unit on the right (minutes). Therefore, the conversion factor for time units must convert minutes to hours.

$$\frac{X \text{ mL}}{1 \text{ hour}} = \frac{15 \text{ mL}}{\cancel{\text{minute}}} \times \frac{60 \ \cancel{\text{minutes}}}{1 \text{ hour}}$$

$$\frac{X \text{ mL}}{1 \text{ hour}} = \frac{15 \text{ mL} \times 60}{1 \text{ hour}}$$

$$\frac{X \text{ mL}}{1 \text{ hour}} = \frac{900 \text{ mL}}{1 \text{ hour}}$$

Therefore, the amount of fluid delivered in one hour at the rate of 15 mL/minute is 900 milliliters.

Volume delivered in 8 hours at a rate of 15 mL/minute:

$$\frac{X \text{ mL}}{8 \text{ hours}} = \frac{15 \text{ mL}}{\text{minute}} \times \frac{60 \text{ minutes}}{1 \text{ hour}}$$

As in one of the previous example problems, the time units in the denominator do not agree, and therefore, the conversion factor must be used to convert minutes to hours.

$$\frac{X \text{ mL}}{8 \text{ hours}} = \frac{15 \text{ mL}}{\cancel{\text{minute}}} \times \frac{60 \; \cancel{\text{minutes}}}{1 \text{ hour}}$$

$$\frac{X \text{ mL}}{8 \text{ hours}} = \frac{15 \text{ mL} \times 60}{1 \text{ hour}}$$

$$\frac{X \text{ mL}}{8 \text{ hours}} = \frac{900 \text{ mL}}{1 \text{ hour}}$$

The time units in both denominators are expressed in hours, but the denominators still don't quite agree because the fraction on the right tells us how many milliliters passed in 1 hour, and we want to know how many passed in *8 hours*. Therefore, we need to convert 1 hour to 8 hours by multiplying the fraction on the right by 8/8.

$$\frac{\text{X mL}}{8 \text{ hours}} = \frac{900 \text{ mL}}{1 \text{ hour}} \times \frac{8}{8}$$

$$\frac{\text{X mL}}{8 \text{ hours}} = \frac{7200 \text{ mL}}{8 \text{ hours}}$$

AN ALTERNATIVE WAY TO DETERMINE RATE OR TOTAL VOLUME

Another way of setting up the problem to determine the rate or total volume using the cancel-out method is to arrange all the knowns and conversion factors as a multiplication series on one side of the equation so that all units cancel out leaving just the unit used for the Unknown. This alternative method follows the same template illustrated in the previous example problems, but allows the problem to be set up as one long step instead of a series of smaller steps.

UNKNOWN = KNOWN VALUE × CONVERSION FACTOR #1 ×
CONVERSION FACTOR #2 × CONVERSION FACTOR #3

To calculate an Unknown flow rate given a
known drip rate, the calibration of the IV
set (drip to mL conversion) and any necessary time unit conversions (seconds to minutes, etc.), we can use the following template:

UNKNOWN RATE =
(VOL/TIME)

DRIP RATE × DRIP-TO-ML CONVERSION × TIME CONVERSION
(GTT/TIME)   (ML/GTT)   (TIME UNIT/TIME UNIT)

Let's use an example to illustrate this.
Given a drip rate of 200 gtt/2 minutes, a
calibration on the IV set of 10 gtt/mL, and
the need to determine what the rate is in
milliliters per second, the problem would
be set up in such a way that everything
would cancel out except milliliters in the
numerator and seconds in the denominator.

$$\frac{mL}{sec} = \frac{200 \text{ gtt}}{2 \text{ min}} \times \frac{1 \text{ mL}}{10 \text{ gtt}} \times \frac{1 \text{ min}}{60 \text{ sec}}$$

$$\frac{mL}{sec} = \frac{200 \,\cancel{\text{gtt}}}{2 \,\cancel{\text{min}}} \times \frac{1 \text{ mL}}{10 \,\cancel{\text{gtt}}} \times \frac{1 \,\cancel{\text{min}}}{60 \text{ sec}}$$

$$\frac{mL}{sec} = \frac{200 \times 1 \text{ mL} \times 1}{2 \times 10 \times 60 \text{ sec}}$$

$$\frac{mL}{sec} = \frac{200 \text{ mL}}{1200 \text{ sec}}$$

$$\frac{mL}{sec} = \frac{0.167 \text{ mL}}{sec}$$

In order to calculate the total volume given the drip rate, IV set calibration, and amount of time for the drip to continue, the equation would be set up so all units cancel out leaving just a volume measurement.

UNKNOWN VOLUME = TIME × TIME CONVERSION × DRIP RATE ×
    (VOLUME)   (TIME UNIT/TIME UNIT) (gtt/TIME)

DRIP-TO-mL CONVERSION
    (mL/gtt)

If we had a drip rate of 5 drips every 10 seconds through an IV set that was calibrated for 60 gtt/mL and this ran for 2 hours, what volume of fluid would have been delivered to the animal?

Volume = 2 hours ×

$$\frac{3600 \text{ seconds}}{1 \text{ hour}} \times \frac{5 \text{ gtt}}{10 \text{ sec}} \times \frac{1 \text{ mL}}{60 \text{ gtt}}$$

Volume = 2 ~~hours~~ ×

$$\frac{3600 \text{ \sout{seconds}}}{1 \text{ \sout{hour}}} \times \frac{5 \text{ \sout{gtt}}}{10 \text{ \sout{sec}}} \times \frac{1 \text{ mL}}{60 \text{ \sout{gtt}}}$$

$$\text{Volume} = \frac{2 \times 3600 \times 5 \times 1 \text{ mL}}{1 \times 10 \times 60}$$

$$\text{Volume} = \frac{36000 \text{ mL}}{600}$$

Volume = 60 mL

Regardless of which method you use to calculate fluid rates for IV infusion, you need to know how to convert from drips to milliliters, from a rate expressed as drips/time unit to milliliters/time unit, and rates from one time unit to another.

SETTING AND ADJUSTING THE IV INFUSION RATE

Being able to determine a given flow rate by observation and calculation is the first step in setting or adjusting the IV infusion rate in order to deliver a set amount of medication at the correct rate. If the infusion rate is too fast, too much drug will be delivered too soon, and drug concentrations in the body may exceed the therapeutic range resulting in toxic side effects. If the infusion rate is too slow, drug concentrations may not achieve therapeutic concentrations and therefore the drug may not be very effective.

To set or adjust the infusion rate to

deliver a given volume of drug in a set period of time, we need three pieces of information:

1. The volume of liquid to be delivered
2. How much time we have to deliver the drug
3. Calibration of the IV administration set (gtt per milliliter)

The rates calculated in these types of problems are expressed as X volume (drips or milliliters) per time (usually minutes or seconds). Once the delivery rate for the fluids is calculated, we would adjust the clamps on the IV tubing to set the observed drip rate to approximate the calculated rate of infusion.

Once again we use the standard template for these type of problems, then we identify specific types of conversion factors that we are going to need to use to arrive at a solution.

UNKNOWN = KNOWN VALUE × CONVERSION FACTOR #1
× CONVERSION FACTOR #2 × CONVERSION FACTOR #3

Our Unknown is the infusion rate (volume/time), the known value is the volume of fluid that needs to be delivered in the specified time span (volume/time), and the conversion factors are going to include any time conversions (e.g., seconds to minutes), volume conversions (mL to liters), and the IV tubing calibration (gtt/mL). Remember, the key to setting up the equation properly is to have all units cancel out leaving only the units used for the Unknown.

Here is an example of how to set up this type of problem. You have been told that a dog needs 3.6 liters of intravenous fluid (or drug dissolved in a total of 3.6 liters of intravenous fluids) in the next 8 hours. The IV infusion set is calibrated for 10 drops per mL. Determine the needed drip rate, expressed as drips per 30 seconds, that will deliver the total volume of fluid within the 8-hour period of time.

UNKNOWN = KNOWN VALUE × CONVERSION FACTOR #1
× CONVERSION FACTOR #2 × CONVERSION FACTOR #3

$$\text{DRIP RATE} = \frac{\text{VOLUME TO BE DELIVERED}}{\text{TIME TO DELIVER IT}}$$

× VOLUME CONVERSION × IV SET CALIBRATION

$$\frac{X \text{ gtt}}{30 \text{ seconds}} = \frac{3.6 \text{ liter}}{8 \text{ hour}} \times$$

$$\frac{1 \text{ hour}}{3600 \text{ seconds}} \times \frac{1000 \text{ mL}}{1 \text{ liter}} \times \frac{10 \text{ gtt}}{1 \text{ mL}}$$

$$\frac{X \text{ gtt}}{30 \text{ seconds}} = \frac{3.6 \text{ liter}}{8 \text{ hour}} \times$$

$$\frac{1 \text{ hour}}{3600 \text{ seconds}} \times \frac{1000 \text{ mL}}{1 \text{ liter}} \times \frac{10 \text{ gtt}}{1 \text{ mL}}$$

$$\frac{X \text{ gtt}}{30 \text{ seconds}} = \frac{3.6 \times 1 \times 1000 \times 10 \text{ gtt}}{8 \times 3600 \text{ seconds} \times 1 \times 1}$$

$$\frac{X \text{ gtt}}{30 \text{ seconds}} = \frac{36000 \text{ gtt}}{28800 \text{ seconds}}$$

$$\frac{X \text{ gtt}}{30 \text{ seconds}} = \frac{1.25 \text{ gtt}}{\text{second}}$$

The result of the calculation is that 1.25 drips per second will deliver the 3.6 liters of fluid in 8 hours. But the question asked was for the drip rate in drips per *30 seconds*. Therefore, we have to multiply the right side of the equation by 30/30 in order to determine the drip rate expressed as number of drips per 30 seconds.

$$\frac{X \text{ gtt}}{30 \text{ seconds}} = \frac{1.25 \text{ gtt}}{\text{second}}$$

$$\frac{X \text{ gtt}}{30 \text{ seconds}} = \frac{1.25 \text{ gtt}}{\text{second}} \times \frac{30}{30}$$

$$\frac{X \text{ gtt}}{30 \text{ seconds}} = \frac{37.5 \text{ gtt}}{30 \text{ seconds}}$$

The 37.5 drips can be rounded either up to 38 drips or down to 37 drips without significantly affecting the overall infusion rate.

DETERMINING THE AMOUNT OF TIME FOR DRIP RATE OBSERVATION

In each of the example problems above, the time unit during which we were to count drips was specified in the problem (e.g., X drips in 30 seconds). Generally, this time unit will not be defined when calculating the drip rate to deliver a set volume of fluid within a specified period of time. Therefore, it is helpful to identify a reasonable period of time to count drips that also provides an accurate representation of the desired infusion rate.

The easiest way to determine a convenient time frame for counting drips is to use the calculated number of drips *per second* and apply that to several possible time frames. Suppose the calculated drip rate to deliver the IV fluid at the proper infusion rate was determined to be 0.35 drips per second. The number of drips for different time frames is easily calculated:

For 10 seconds:

$$\frac{\text{X gtt}}{10 \text{ seconds}} = \frac{0.35 \text{ gtt}}{\text{second}} \times \frac{10}{10}$$

$$\frac{X \text{ gtt}}{10 \text{ seconds}} = \frac{3.5 \text{ gtt}}{10 \text{ seconds}}$$

For 20 seconds:

$$\frac{X \text{ gtt}}{20 \text{ seconds}} = \frac{0.35 \text{ gtt}}{\text{second}} \times \frac{20}{20}$$

$$\frac{X \text{ gtt}}{20 \text{ seconds}} = \frac{7 \text{ gtt}}{20 \text{ seconds}}$$

We wrote out the steps in the process simply for clarification. The easiest way to determine multiple time frames is simply to take the number of drips in 1 second and multiply it by the number of seconds for your possible observation time frame.

$0.35 \text{ gtt} \times 5 \quad = \quad 1.75 \text{ gtt in 5 seconds}$

$0.35 \text{ gtt} \times 10 = \quad 3.5 \text{ gtt in 10 seconds}$

$0.35 \text{ gtt} \times 15 = \quad 5.25 \text{ gtt in 15 seconds}$

$0.35 \text{ gtt} \times 20 = \quad 7 \text{ gtt in 20 seconds}$

$0.35 \text{ gtt} \times 30 = \quad 10.5 \text{ gtt in 30 seconds}$

Looking over the possible choices, the "7 drips in 20 seconds" seems the most reasonable, because it involves a whole number of drips (no rounding required) and the time frame for observation is reasonably short.

SECTION I
PRACTICE PROBLEMS
(Answers are at the end of the chapter.)

1) For each of the following IV set calibrations (gtt/mL) and the observed drip rate, determine the flow in the units listed.

a) 10 gtt/mL 20 drips per minute
= _____ mL/minute

b) 15 gtt/mL 300 drips per minute
= _____ mL/minute

c) 20 gtt/mL 320 drips per minute
= _____ mL/minute

d) 60 gtt/mL 1260 drips per minute
= _____ mL/minute

e) 10 gtt/mL 1 drip per second
= _____ mL/minute

f) 20 gtt/mL 2 drips per second
= _____ mL/minute

g) 60 gtt/mL 3 drips per second
= _____ mL/minute

h) 20 gtt/mL 3 drips every 6 seconds
   = _____ mL/minute

i) 15 gtt/mL 15 drips every 10 seconds
   = _____ mL/minute

j) 60 gtt/mL 30 drips every 15 seconds
   = _____ mL/minute

2) For each of the following IV tubing calibrations, the observed drip rate, and the length of time, determine how many milliliters are delivered in the stated length of time.

a) 10 gtt/mL 2 drips per second for
   15 minutes = _____ mL

b) 20 gtt/mL 1 drip per second for
   10 minutes = _____ mL

c) 60 gtt/mL 10 drips every 20 seconds
   for
   20 minutes = _____ mL

d) 15 gtt/mL 30 drips every 45 seconds
   for 15 minutes = _____ mL

e) 20 gtt/mL 2 drips every 5 seconds for
   12 minutes = _____ mL

f) 60 gtt/mL 12 drips every 5 seconds for
   30 minutes = _____ mL

3. For each of the following situations, determine the drip rate (X drips per Y seconds) given the volume of drug or fluids that needs to be infused, the amount of time to infuse the volume, and the calibration of the IV set.

a) 810 mL, 6 hours, 20 gtt/mL: _____ drops every _____ seconds

b) 180 mL, 12 hours, 60 gtt/mL: _____ drops every _____ seconds

c) 768 mL, 4 hours, 15 gtt/mL: _____ drops every _____ seconds

d) 162 mL, 6 hours, 20 gtt/mL: _____ drops every _____ seconds

e) 0.9 liters, 12 hours, 60 gtt/mL: _____ drops every _____ seconds

f) 4.5 liters, 15 hours, 20 gtt/mL: _____ drops every _____ seconds

SECTION II CALCULATING INFUSION RATES WHEN ADDING DRUGS TO IV FLUIDS

Often drugs may be added to the intravenous fluids as a means of infusing a drug over a set period of time. If we are to determine the infusion rate, we need to determine the volume of drug that is to be added to the volume of IV fluids. The volume of drug is determined using the calculated dose for the particular animal (mg of drug) and the drug concentration within the vial (mg of drug /mL of liquid). See Chapter 7 for more details on this calculation procedure. Once the volume of drug is determined, it must be summed with the volume of intravenous fluids in the bag or bottle to determine the total volume that must be delivered over time.

Here is an example. An animal needs 25 mg of drug to be infused over 4 hours. The concentration of drug in the vial is 10 mg per mL. The IV fluid bag into which the drug is going to be added is 500 mL. The IV infusion set has a drip rate of 20 gtt/mL. What drip rate is going to be needed in order to deliver the drug in 4 hours?

Although this may seem like a lot of information to put into an equation at one time, it becomes much more manageable when you construct the equation one piece at a time. Start first with the volume of drug to be added.

UNKNOWN = KNOWN VALUE × CONVERSION FACTOR

DRUG VOLUME = DRUG DOSE (MG) × CONCENTRATION (MG/ML)

$$X \text{ mL} = 25 \text{ mg drug} \times \frac{1 \text{ mL liquid in vial}}{10 \text{ mg drug}}$$

$$X \text{ mL} = 25 \; \cancel{\text{mg drug}} \times \frac{1 \text{ mL liquid in vial}}{10 \; \cancel{\text{mg drug}}}$$

$$X \text{ mL} = \frac{25 \times 1 \text{ mL}}{10}$$

$$X \text{ mL} = 2.5 \text{ mL}$$

Therefore, 2.5 mL of drug will be withdrawn from the vial and added to the 500 mL of IV fluids to give a total volume of 502.5 milliliters to be delivered in 4 hours. This would be expressed as an infusion rate of :

$$\frac{502.5 \text{ mL}}{4 \text{ hours}}$$

The drip rate is then determined as it was in Section I.

UNKNOWN = KNOWN VALUE × CONVERSION FACTOR #1 × CONVERSION FACTOR #2 × CONVERSION FACTOR #3

DRIP RATE =

<u>VOLUME TO BE DELIVERED</u> × TIME CONVERSION ×   TIME TO DELIVER IT

VOLUME CONVERSION × IV SET CALIBRATION

$$\frac{X \text{ gtt}}{\text{second}} =$$

$$\frac{502.5 \text{ mL}}{4 \text{ hours}} \times \frac{1 \text{hour}}{3600 \text{ seconds}} \times \frac{20 \text{ gtt}}{1 \text{ mL}}$$

$$\frac{X \text{ gtt}}{\text{second}} =$$

$$\frac{502.5 \, \cancel{\text{mL}}}{4 \, \cancel{\text{hours}}} \times \frac{1 \cancel{\text{hour}}}{3600 \text{ seconds}} \times \frac{20 \text{ gtt}}{1 \, \cancel{\text{mL}}}$$

$$\frac{X \text{ gtt}}{\text{second}} = \frac{502.5 \times 1 \times 20 \text{ drips}}{4 \times 3600 \times 1}$$

$$\frac{X \text{ gtt}}{\text{second}} = \frac{10050 \text{ drips}}{14400 \text{ seconds}}$$

$$\frac{X \text{ gtt}}{\text{second}} = \frac{0.698 \text{ drips}}{\text{second}}$$

Given the calculated drip date per second, it is easy to determine the drip rate expressed as drips per 5, 10, 15, or 20 seconds.

$$\frac{0.698 \text{ drips}}{\text{second}} = \frac{3.49}{5 \text{ seconds}} = \frac{6.98}{10 \text{ seconds}} =$$

$$\frac{10.47}{15 \text{ seconds}} = \frac{13.96}{20 \text{ seconds}}$$

By selecting the time frames in which the number is closest to a whole drip, we can set our drip rate to either 7 drips in 10 seconds or 14 drips in 20 seconds.

To summarize, when calculating a drip rate for infusion of a drug in IV fluids within a set period of time, the steps would be:

1. Determine the *volume* of drug to be added to the fluid
2. Determine the total volume of IV fluid and drug to be delivered by the set time frame
3. Determine the drip rate to deliver the total fluid

SECTION II
PRACTICE PROBLEMS
(Answers are at the end of the chapter.)

1. Telazol® tiletamine (Figure 9.2) is going to be infused into a zoo animal at a dose of 350 mg over 1 hour. The drug is going to be diluted in 1 liter of IV fluids. Determine the drip rate for an IV administration set calibrated to 10 gtt/1 mL.

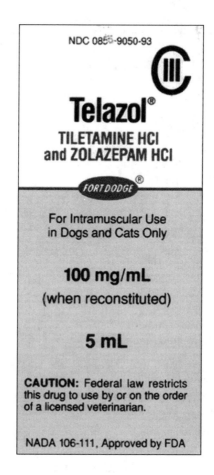

Figure 9.2 Telazol® (tiletamine)

2. For each of the following situations, determine the drip rate (X drips per Y sec-

onds) given the drug dose, the drug concentration, the volume of fluids into which the drug volume will be added, the amount of time to infuse the volume, and the calibration of the IV set.

a) 125 mg, 50 mg/mL, 500 mL, 5 hours, 20 gtt/mL

b) 350 mg, 25 mg/mL, 1 liter, 12 hours, 60 gtt/mL

c) 48.5 mg, 10 mg/mL, 300 mL, 1 1/2 hours, 15 gtt/mL

d) 1 gram, 100 mg/mL, 1/2 liter, 6 hours, 10 gtt/mL

e) 2 grains, 480 mg/mL, 1/4 liter, 3 hour, 20 gtt/mL

SECTION III
CALCULATING STOP TIMES FOR INFUSION RATES

In the previous section we learned how to calculate the drip rate given a volume that needed to be delivered by a prescribed time. However, commonly the *infusion rate* will be prescribed, and from that the amount of time for the infusion needs to be determined so that the IV infusion can be stopped, the IV line flushed, additional medication given, or backflow of blood into the IV set prevented.

In this situation we use the same basic formula as with the previous problem examples, except that now the Unknown X is the time for the infusion, the known value is the volume to be delivered, and the conversion factor is the infusion rate (in time units per volume).

UNKNOWN = KNOWN VALUE × CONVERSION FACTOR

TIME FOR THE INFUSION = VOLUME TO BE DELIVERED ×
VOLUME CONVERSION × TIME CONVERSION ×
INFUSION RATE (time/vol)

Notice how the infusion rate is listed in this formula as *time unit per volume.* Because our answer is a time unit, we need to have a time unit in the numerator of our equation. Therefore, this arrangement will allow all the units to cancel appropriately leaving just the time unit.

Notice that the IV administration set calibration is not used in this equation. The reason for this is that most prescribed infusion rates will be listed as milliliters per minute, or milligrams of drug per minute (for which the volume of drug would need to be determined).

Let's illustrate how to set up this type of problem using an example. If we need to deliver 1 liter of fluids at a rate of 2 mL per

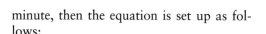
minute, then the equation is set up as follows:

$$X \text{ hours} = 1 \text{ liter} \times$$

$$\frac{1000 \text{ mL}}{1 \text{ liter}} \times \frac{1 \text{ hour}}{60 \text{ minutes}} \times \frac{1 \text{ minute}}{2 \text{ mL}}$$

$$X \text{ hours} = 1 \, \cancel{\text{liter}} \times$$

$$\frac{1000 \, \cancel{\text{mL}}}{1 \, \cancel{\text{liter}}} \times \frac{1 \text{ hour}}{60 \, \cancel{\text{minutes}}} \times \frac{1 \, \cancel{\text{minute}}}{2 \, \cancel{\text{mL}}}$$

$$X \text{ hours} = \frac{1 \times 1000 \times 1 \text{ hour} \times 1}{1 \times 60 \times 2}$$

$$X \text{ hours} = \frac{1000 \text{ hours}}{120}$$

$$X \text{ hours} = 8.33 \text{ hours}$$

Therefore, for the volume prescribed and the infusion rate prescribed, the fluids will be delivered 8.33 hours after the infusion is started.

To prevent confusion for the veterinary technician who has to carry out these orders, we would calculate the scheduled stop time for the infusion and write it as a certain hour and minute. For example, after starting the infusion, the clinician might write: "The infusion should be stopped at 5:45 P.M."

THE 24-HOUR CLOCK

In the example problem above, confusion can sometimes occur if drug orders are given to "Stop the infusion at 12:00 P.M." (is that noon or midnight?) or "at 7:35" (is it 7:35 in the morning or evening?). For that reason, some medical institutions issue start/stop orders for infusions according to a 24-hour clock as opposed to using the A.M. and P.M. designations.

The 24-hour clock starts at 00:00 (zero hours and zero minutes) at midnight and runs to 23:59 (23 hours and 59 minutes after midnight). The first twelve hours (morning) on the 24-hour clock are the same as the 12 hour clock, but the second 12 hours on the 24-hour clock add 12 to the hour value. Examples are shown below.

A.M. P.M.	24-hour clock
12:00 A.M.	0:00
1:01 A.M.	1:01
9:56 A.M.	9:56
12:00 P.M. (noon)	12:00
1:00 P.M.	13:00
6:26 P.M.	18:26
11:24 P.M.	23:24

The veterinary professional should be able to use both methods of describing time.

CONVERTING TOTAL INFUSION TIME

The veterinary professional also needs to know how to convert total infusion time to 12-hour and 24-hour clock stop times. In the example problem above, the stop time was calculated to be 8.33 hours after the infusion was started. One of the mistakes made in calculating the actual stop time (e.g., 6:45, 18:45, etc.) is that the 0.33 is interpreted as "33 minutes" instead of 0.33 hours. Remember that 0.33 hours is equivalent to 20 minutes, not 33 minutes:

$$X \text{ minutes} = 0.33 \text{ hours} \times \frac{60 \text{ minutes}}{1 \text{ hour}}$$

$$X \text{ minutes} = 0.33 \, \cancel{\text{hours}} \times \frac{60 \text{ minutes}}{1 \, \cancel{\text{hour}}}$$

$$X \text{ minutes} = \frac{0.33 \times 60 \text{ minutes}}{1}$$

$$X \text{ minutes} = 20 \text{ minutes}$$

Therefore, the infusion is stopped 8 hours and 20 minutes after it has been started. If the start time for this infusion was 1:15 P.M. (13:15), then the stop time can be calculated as follows:

Step 1. Add the number of minutes together.

Step 2. If the minutes are greater than 60, subtract 60 from the total minutes, "give" 1 to the hours, and use the remainder for the minutes value.

Step 3. Add the hours together including any "given" from the minutes.

Step 4. If the hours are greater than 24 (12 for the 12-hour clock) then subtract 24 from the hours (12 from the hours for the 12-hour clock) and use the remainder for the hours value.

For the 12-hour clock:

Start time: 1:15 = 1 hour and 15 minutes

Calculated infusion time: 8 hours and 20 minutes

Step 1: 15 minutes + 20 minutes = 35 minutes

Step 2: Check to see if greater than 60 minutes. 35 minutes < 60 minutes.

Step 3: 1 hour + 8 hours = 9 hours

Step 4: Check to see if hours are greater than 12 hours. 9 hours < 12 hours.

The stop time is 9:35 P.M.

For the 24-hour clock:

Start time: 13:15 = 13 hours and 15 minutes

Calculated infusion time: 8 hours and 20 minutes

Step 1: 15 minutes + 20 minutes = 35 minutes

Step 2: Check to see if greater than 60 minutes. 35 minutes < 60 minutes.

Step 3: 13 hours + 8 hours = 21 hours

Step 4: Check to see if hours are greater than 24 hours. 21 hours < 24 hours.

The stop time is 21:35 P.M.

The following calculation illustrates how a stop time might be calculated for the 8 hour 20 minute infusion if the start time were 22:43 (10:43 P.M.) hours.

For the 12-hour clock:

Start time: 10:43 = 10 hours and 43 minutes

Calculated infusion time: 8 hours and 20 minutes

Step 1: 43 minutes + 20 minutes = 63 minutes

Step 2: Check to see if greater than 60 minutes. It is. 63 − 60 = 3

Add 1 to the hours and use the 3 for the minutes value.

Step 3: 10 hours + 8 hours + 1 hour = 19 hours

Step 4: Check to see if hours are greater than 12 hours. It is. 19 − 12 = 7

Change the P.M. to A.M.

The stop time is 7:03 A.M.

For 24-hour clock:

Start time: 22:43 = 22 hours and 43 minutes

Calculated infusion time: 8 hours and 20 minutes

Step 1: 43 minutes + 20 minutes = 63 minutes

Step 2: Check to see if greater than 60 minutes. It is. 63 − 60 = 3.

Add 1 to the hours and use the 3 for the minutes value.

Step 3: 22 hours + 8 hours + 1 hour = 31 hours

Step 4: Check to see if hours are greater than 24 hours. It is. 31 − 24 = 7

The stop time is 07:03 hour.

SECTION III
PRACTICE PROBLEMS
(Answers are at the end of the chapter.)

1. Given the following times on the 12-hour clock, convert them to the 24-hour clock designations.

a) 1:35 A.M.   d) 3:15 P.M.

b) 8:00 P.M.   e) 10:25 P.M.

c) 11:45 A.M.   f) 7:54 P.M.

2. Given the volume of fluid to be delivered and the infusion rate, determine how many hours and minutes it will take to deliver the fluid.

a) 250 mL, 2 mL/min

b) 1500 mL, 15 mL/min

c) 2 liters, 5 mL/min

d) 3.6 liters, 12 mL/min

e) 5.25 liters, 0.5 mL/second

f) 880 mL, 4 mL/min

3. Given the volume of fluid to be delivered, the infusion rate, and the start time, determine the stop time in both 12- and 24-hour clock nomenclature.

a) 450 mL, 2 mL/min, 03:10

b) 1200 mL, 5 mL/min, 10:51 A.M.

c) 900 mL, 3 mL/min, 13:35

d) 2.2 liter, 4 mL/min, 19:21

e) 1.15 liter, 2.5 mL/min, 23:44

f) 0.035 liter, 0.125 mL/min, 03:59

ANSWERS FOR PRACTICE PROBLEMS

SECTION I

1) a) $\dfrac{20 \text{ gtt}}{\text{min}} \times \dfrac{1 \text{ mL}}{10 \text{ gtt}} = \dfrac{20 \text{ mL}}{10 \text{ min}} =$

2 mL/minute

b) 20 mL/minute

c) 16 mL/minute

d) 21 mL/minute

e) $\dfrac{1 \text{ gtt}}{\text{sec}} \times \dfrac{60 \text{ seconds}}{1 \text{ minute}} \times \dfrac{1 \text{ mL}}{10 \text{ gtt}} =$

$\dfrac{60 \text{ mL}}{10 \text{ min}} = 6 \text{ mL/minute}$

f) 6 mL/minute

g) 3 mL/minute

h) $\dfrac{3 \text{ gtt}}{6 \text{ sec}} \times \dfrac{60 \text{ seconds}}{1 \text{ minute}} \times \dfrac{1 \text{ mL}}{20 \text{ gtt}}$

$= \dfrac{180 \text{ mL}}{120 \text{ min}} = 1.5 \text{ mL/minute}$

i) 6 mL/minute

j) 2 mL/minute

2) a) $15 \text{ min} \times \dfrac{60 \text{ sec}}{1 \text{ minute}} \times \dfrac{2 \text{ gtt}}{\text{sec}} \times \dfrac{1 \text{ mL}}{10 \text{ gtt}}$

$= \dfrac{1800 \text{ mL}}{10} = 180 \text{ mL}$

    b) 30 mL

    c) 10 mL

    d) 40 mL

    e) 14.4 mL

    f) 72 mL

3) a) 15 drops every 20 seconds

    b) 5 drops every 20 seconds

    c) 4 drops every 5 seconds

    d) 3 drops every 20 seconds

    e) 25 drops every 20 seconds

    f) 25 drops every 15 seconds

SECTION II

1) $350 \text{ mg} \times \dfrac{1 \text{ mL}}{100 \text{ mg}} = 3.5 \text{ mL}$

$3.5 \text{ mL} + 1000 \text{ mL (1 liter)} = 1003.5 \text{ mL}$

$$\dfrac{1003.5 \text{ mL}}{1 \text{ hour}} \times \dfrac{1 \text{ hour}}{3600 \text{ sec}} \times \dfrac{10 \text{ gtt}}{1 \text{ mL}} =$$

$$\frac{2.788 \text{ drips}}{\text{sec}} = \frac{14 \text{ drips}}{5 \text{ sec}}$$

2) a) 6 drips every 10 seconds

b) 7 drips every 5 seconds or 14 every 10 seconds

c) 17 drips every 20 seconds

d) 7 drips every 30 seconds

e) 9 drips every 20 seconds

SECTION III

1. a) 01:35   d) 15:15

b) 20:00   e) 22:25

c) 11:45   f) 19:54

2. a) 125 minutes = 2 hours, 5 minutes

b) 100 minutes = 1 hour, 40 minutes

c) 400 minutes = 6 hours, 40 minutes

d) 300 minutes = 5 hours

e) 10,500 seconds = 175 minutes = 2 hours, 55 minutes

f) 220 minutes = 3 hours, 40 minutes

3. a) 225 minute infusion 6:55 A.M.
   3 hours, 45 minutes 06:55

   b) 240 minute infusion 2:51 P.M.
   4 hours, 0 minutes 14:51

   c) 300 minute infusion 6:35 P.M.
   5 hours, 0 minutes 18:35

   d) 550 minute infusion 4:31 A.M.
   9 hours, 10 minutes 04:31

   e) 460 minute infusion 7:24 A.M.
   7 hours, 40 minutes 07:24

   f) 280 minute infusion 8:39 A.M.
   4 hours, 40 minutes 08:39

CHAPTER 9 PROBLEMS

1) For each of the following IV set calibrations (gtt/mL) and the observed drip rate, determine the flow in the units listed.

a) 20 gtt/mL 30 drips per minute
= _____ mL/minute

b) 10 gtt/mL 230 drips per minute
=_____ mL/minute

c) 60 gtt/mL 240 drips per minute
=_____ mL/minute

d) 10 gtt/mL 20 drips every 30 seconds
=_____ mL/minute

e) 20 gtt/mL 5 drips every 10 seconds
= _____ mL/minute

f) 60 gtt/mL 25 drips every 15 seconds
= _____ mL/minute

g) 10 gtt/mL 7 drips every 10 seconds
=_____ mL/minute

h) 15 gtt/mL 25 drips every 20 seconds
=_____ mL/minute

i) 60 gtt/mL 30 drips every 15 seconds
=_____ mL/minute

j) 20 gtt/mL 2 drips every 5 seconds
=_____ mL/minute

2) For each of the following IV tubing calibrations, the observed drip rate, and the length of time, determine how many milliliters are delivered in the stated length of time.

a) 10 gtt/mL 1 drip per second
5 minutes =_____ mL

b) 20 gtt/mL 2 drips per second
30 minutes =_____ mL

c) 15 gtt/mL 8 drips every 20 seconds
25 minutes =_____ mL

d) 60 gtt/mL 37 drips every 45 seconds
40 minutes =_____ mL

e) 20 gtt/mL 3 drips every 15 seconds
1 hour   =_____ mL

f) 15 gtt/mL 22 drips every 10 seconds
3.5 hours =_____ mL

3) For each of the following situations determine the drip rate (X drips per Y seconds), given the volume of drug or fluids that needs to be infused, the amount of time to infuse the volume, and the calibration of the IV set.

a) 750 mL, 2.5 hours, 15 gtt/mL_____ drops every _____ seconds

b) 200 mL, 10 hours, 60 gtt/mL_____ drops every _____ seconds

c) 120 mL, 1 hour, 20 gtt/mL_____ drops every _____ seconds

d) 1500 mL, 7.5 hours, 15 gtt/mL_____
drops every _____ seconds

e) 4 liters, 10 hours, 15 gtt/mL_____
drops every _____ seconds

f) 1.25 liters, 15 hours, 10 gtt/mL_____
drops every _____ seconds

4) For each of the following situations determine what the drip rate (X drips per Y seconds) given the drug dose, the drug concentration, the volume of fluids into which the drug volume will be added, the amount of time to infuse the volume, and the calibration of the IV set.

a) 600 mg, 200 mg/mL, 100 mL, 4.25 hours, 20 gtt/mL

b) 250 mg, 25 mg/mL, 1 liter, 12 hours, 10 gtt/mL

c) 4.8 grams, 40 mg/mL, 100 mL, 5 1/2 hours, 15 gtt/mL

d) 450 mg, 5 mg/mL, 1/4 liter, 4 hours, 20 gtt/mL

e) 3 grains, 0.03 grams/mL, 360 mL, 6 hours, 60 gtt/mL

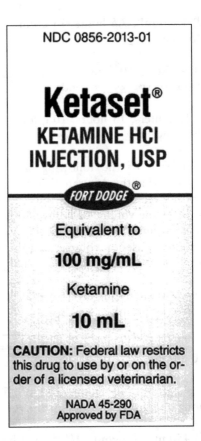

NDC 0856-2013-01

Ketaset®
**KETAMINE HCl
INJECTION, USP**

FORT DODGE ®

Equivalent to

100 mg/mL

Ketamine

10 mL

CAUTION: Federal law restricts this drug to use by or on the order of a licensed veterinarian.

NADA 45-290
Approved by FDA

Figure 9.3 Ketaset® (ketamine)

5) The veterinarian is going to infuse this drug intravenously for 1 hour as part of an anesthetic protocol. He wants to deliver 400 mg total during that period of time. He

is going to use 200 mL of intravenous fluids to dilute the ketamine. The IV administration set is calibrated to 10 gtt per milliliter. What drip rate (X drips per Y seconds) will you use to ensure the proper infusion rate?

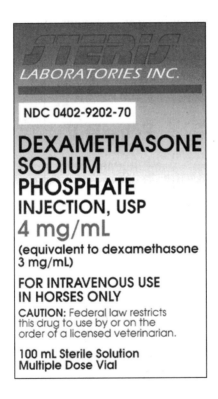

Figure 9.4 Dexamethasone sodium phosphate

6) This drug is going to be infused over the next four hours to help to reduce cerebral swelling from trauma. The total dose delivered will be 110 mg. The drug will be injected into a 1/2 liter IV fluid bag for administration through a 20 gtt/mL IV administration set. What drip rate will deliver this drug at a constant rate over the required time frame?

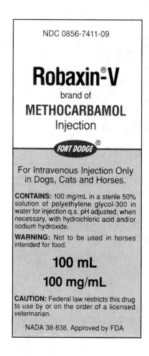

Figure 9.5 Robaxin®-V (methocarbamol)

7) This drug is needed to be delivered over the next 30 minutes. It will be added to a 250 mL IV fluid bottle. The dose this animal is to receive is 250 mg. The IV set is calibrated at 10 gtt/mL. What drip rate should be used to deliver this drug by a 30-minute infusion?

8) You are presented with a 40 lb animal that needs a drug given over 5 hours at a dose of 5 mg/kg. You decide that an infusion with 1 liter of fluids using a 15 gtt/mL IV set will allow you to control the infusion rate fairly accurately. The concentration of drug in the vial is 200 mg/mL. What drip rate (X drips per Y seconds) will you use to deliver this drug over the 5-hour infusion period?

OTHER CALCULATIONS USED BY VETERINARY PROFESSIONALS

Objectives

The student will be able to perform the following:

1. Recognize ratio and proportion formats in literature and convert them to equations for solving problems.

2. Convert between degrees Fahrenheit and degrees Celsius (Centigrade).

3. Translate Roman numerals into numerical values and write Roman numeral representations of numerical values.

In addition to drug dosing calculations, there are other mathematical calculations that many veterinary professionals encounter in their occupations. This chapter will introduce some of these calculations for familiarity and reference.

SECTION I RATIOS AND PROPORTIONS— SOME ADDITIONAL POINTS

Ratios were referred to in previous chapters when utilizing the ratio method for calculating drug doses. Ratios sometimes appear in veterinary literature and are used when drugs are compounded with two or more types of raw materials. Therefore, familiarity with the nomenclature and use of ratios is important.

A ratio is the relationship between two numbers. For example, 100 mg of drug in 1 capsule would produce the ratio of:

100 mg : 1 capsule

The nomenclature used here is sometimes seen in the medical literature. The colon ":" indicates that the item on the left is equivalent to the item on the right. In this case, the 100 mg of drug is equal in drug amount to 1 capsule of that particular drug. We used ratios in the conversion factors throughout this text. Here are some conversion factors represented as ratios using the colon nomenclature:

$$\frac{200 \text{ mg}}{\text{mL}} \text{ drug concentration}$$

200 mg : 1 mL

$$\frac{15 \text{ gtt}}{\text{mL}} \text{ calibration of IV set}$$

15 gtt : 1 mL

$$\frac{0.5 \text{ grain phenobarbital}}{\text{tablet}}$$

0.5 grain : 1 tablet

In the ratio method of calculating dosages, we set up two ratios as fractions, of which one component (either the numerator or denominator) of one fraction was the Unknown X.

$$\frac{X \text{ kg}}{10 \text{ lb}} = \frac{1 \text{ kg}}{2.2 \text{ lb}}$$

There are two ratios contained in this equation:

X kg : 10 lb

1 kg : 2.2 lb

Because the two ratios are mathematically equal to each other, they represent a proportion. When we say that one ratio is proportional to another ratio, we mean that if you multiplied both components of one ratio by a particular number, you would get the second ratio, or vice versa.

The two ratios of kilograms and pounds can be represented as a proportion using the following nomenclature:

X kg : 10 lb : : 1 kg : 2.2 lb

The double set of colon marks "∷" indicates that the two ratios are proportional to each other. To use this mathematical representation of proportion in a calculation, convert it into the fraction form for use with either the ratio method or the cancel-out method. Once in the more familiar fraction equation form, the Unknown X is easily calculated.

SECTION I
PRACTICE PROBLEMS
(Answers are at the end of the chapter.)

1) Write each of the following ratios in fraction form and solve for the Unknown X:

a) 50 mg : 1 tablet ∷ X mg : 5 tablets

b) 100 mg : 1 mL ∷ 400 mg : X mL

c) X grams : 2 capsules ∷ 5 grams : 10 capsules

d) 25 mg : X cc ∷ 300 mg : 480 cc

e) $1.00 : 2 tablets ∷ $ X : 16 tablets

f) 10 gtt : 2.5 mL ∷ 240 gtt : X mL

SECTION II CONVERTING TEMPERATURE VALUES BETWEEN FAHRENHEIT AND CELSIUS

Increasingly, body temperatures of veterinary patients are written in literature and medical records as degrees Celsius (also called degrees Centigrade), as opposed to the more familiar Fahrenheit scale commonly used in the United States. Because of the increasing use of the Celsius scale, the veterinary professional should become familiar with how to accurately convert from the Fahrenheit to the Celsius (Centigrade) scale, and vice versa.

The Fahrenheit scale uses $32°$ F as the point at which water freezes, and $212°$ F as the temperature at which water boils. The Celsius has taken these two end points and made them $0°$ C for water freezing and $100°$ C for water boiling.

Before we give the formula for converting between these two scales, a brief look at the proportions of these scales will help in correctly remembering and applying the appropriate formula.

Notice the difference between $32°$ F and $212°$ F is 180 degrees whereas the difference between these two points on the Celsius scale is only 100 degrees ($100°$ C – $0°$ C). It would stand to reason that in converting from the more expansive scale of Fahrenheit (expansive in terms of number of degrees between freezing and boiling) to the more compact scale of Celsius, we would have to multiply the larger Fahrenheit value by some factor that would make the Fahrenheit number proportionally "smaller" or less in value.

The ratio of number of Celsius increments between freezing and boiling of water to Fahrenheit is:

$$\frac{100 \text{ increments}}{180 \text{ increments}}$$

This reduces to the fraction

$$\frac{5}{9}$$

This fraction plays a key role in converting from Fahrenheit to Celsius. The reciprocal, 9/5, is used in converting Celsius to Fahrenheit.

The other key factor that enters into these temperature conversions incorporates the differences between the temperature on both scales at which water freezes. If the freezing point is considered the baseline of the scale, it is necessary to orient both scales to a common value for the baseline. The Fahrenheit scale's baseline is at 32° F, whereas the Celsius scale baseline is 0° C. Therefore, in making a comparison (or a conversion) from Fahrenheit to Celsius, we need to subtract 32 from any Fahrenheit value. If we subtract 32 from the freezing point of 32° F, we get a value of zero, which corresponds to the freezing point of the Celsius scale.

By remembering to appropriately use the reducing fraction 5/9 or the expanding fraction 9/5 and to subtract or add 32 points to reflect the difference between the Fahrenheit and Celsius scales' baselines for freezing, we can make sense out of the formulas for converting between the two scales.

Celsius (Centigrade) temperature = (F − 32) × 5/9

Fahrenheit temperature = (C × 9/5) + 32

For the calculation of Celsius, we first subtract 32 from a Fahrenheit value (this normalizes the Fahrenheit scale to the same baseline as Celsius) then condense the Fahrenheit scale value proportionally to the Celsius scale by multiplying by 5/9.

To convert from the more compact Celsius scale to the more expansive Fahrenheit scale, we first expand the Celsius value by multiplying it by the larger fraction, 9/5. We then reset the baseline to that of the Fahrenheit scale of 32 by adding 32 to the product of the 9/5 multiplication.

Here are some common conversions between the two scales. You should be very familiar with the Celsius (Centigrade) measurements normally used for body temperatures.

Fahrenheit	Celsius (Centigrade)
0	−17.8
32	0
50	10.0
90	32.2
98.6	37.0
100	37.8
100.4	38.0
102.2	39.0
104	40.0

SECTION II
PRACTICE PROBLEMS
(Answers are at the end of the chapter.)

1. For each of the following Fahrenheit values, convert to Celsius (Centigrade).

a) 60° F

b) 90° F

c) 104° F

d) 108° F

2. For each of the following Celsius (Centigrade) values, convert to Fahrenheit.

a) 35° C

b) 42° C

c) 22° C

d) 30° C

SECTION III
ROMAN NUMERAL NOMENCLATURE

Occasionally Roman numeral nomenclature appears in the medical literature. Perhaps the most commonly encountered Roman numerals are on the front of boxes of controlled substance drugs. In this situation, a large C and a Roman numeral indicate the potential for abuse from a C-II designation (most potential for abuse for drugs that can be legally prescribed) to C-V, which are drugs with minimal potential for abuse. C-I drugs are those that have "no legitimate medicinal value," such as LSD, heroin, or crack cocaine.

There are only a few basic characters most commonly used to represent numerical values in the Roman numeral system.

I = 1
V = 5
X = 10
L = 50

$$C = 100$$
$$D = 500$$
$$M = 1000$$
$$\overline{V} = 5000$$

These characters can be used to represent every number from 1 to 9,999.

WRITING ROMAN NUMERALS

To write a Roman numeral to represent a numerical value, first break the numerical value into each of its components, then combine the individual Roman numeral characters to represent each of the values of 10 (e.g., 1, 10, 100, 1000, etc.) starting with the largest factor of 10. For example, to write the Roman numeral to represent the value 1,123, we would first break the numerical value into $1000 + 100 + 10 + 10 + 1 + 1 + 1$. We would then substitute the Roman numeral for each of the components.

$1000 + 100 + 10 + 10 + 1 + 1 + 1$

M   C   X   X   I   I   I

Thus the Roman numeral representation of the numerical value of 1,123 is MCXXIII.

There is an exception to this rule. As you can see, Roman numeral representation of a numerical value can get lengthy! In order to prevent Roman numerals from becoming too cumbersome, the numerical values of 4, 9, 40, 90, 400, and 900 are represented by using two characters, of which the lesser valued character value is *subtracted* from the other. For example, the numerical value "4" is represented in Roman numerals by the character for "1" (I) and "5" (V). The lower-valued character is written to the left and subtracted from the larger-valued character.

IV = 5 − 1 = 4   I is 1, V is 5

IX = 10 − 1 = 9   I is 1, X is 10

XL = 50 −10 = 40   X is 10, L is 50

XC = 100 − 10 = 90   X is 10, C is 100

CD = 500 − 100 = 400 C is 100, D is 500

CM = 1000−100 = 900   C is 100, M is 1000

When reading Roman numerals from left to right, whenever a *lesser-valued* Roman numeral character precedes a larger value, it indicates that the lesser-valued character is to be subtracted from the larger-valued character.

Here is another example of writing a Roman numeral in which some fours and nines are embedded.

2,329 =
1000 + 1000 + 100 + 100 + 100 + 10 +
  M   M   C   C   C   X

10 + (10 − 1)
X   IX

MMCCCXXIX

1,472 =
1000 + (500 − 100) + 50 + 10 + 10 + 1 + 1
  M   CD   L   X   X I I

MCDLXXII

2,149 =
1000 + 1000 + 100 + (50 − 10) + (10 − 1)
  M   M   C   XL   IX

MMCXLIX

READING ROMAN NUMERALS

The numerical values of the Roman numerals are determined by reading the Roman numeral from left to right. The values of each individual Roman numeral are added together to produce the final value.

XV = 10 + 5 = 15   X is 10, V is 5

LII = 50 + 1 + 1 = 52   L is 50, I is 1

CXIII = 100 + 10 + 1 + 1 + 1 = 113

C is 100, X is 10, I is 1

The trickiest part of reading Roman numerals is reading and recognizing the representation of the values of "4" and "9." The following examples illustrate how to read more "complex" Roman numerals.

XXIV = 10 + 10 + (5 − 1) = 20 + 4 = 24

XXXIX = 10 + 10 + 10 + (10 − 1) = 30 + 9 = 39

XLII = (50 − 10) + 1 + 1 = 40 + 2 = 42

XCVIII = (100 − 10) + 5 + 1 + 1 + 1 = 90 + 8 = 98

CDXLIV = (500 − 100) + (50 − 10) + (5 − 1) = 400 + 40 + 4 = 444

MCMXCIX = 1000 + (1000 − 100) + (100 − 10) + (10 − 1) = 1999

By practicing with Roman numerals, the veterinary professional can become familiar with the basic characters and quickly recognize the numeric values represented by strings of Roman numerals.

SECTION III
PRACTICE PROBLEMS
(Answers are at the end of the chapter.)

1. Given the following Roman numerals, write the value for each.

a) XII

b) XXV

c) XLVII

d) LXIV

e) XCIII

f) CXXIX

g) CCCXXXIV

h) MCCXXXVII

i) MCMXXXV

j) MCMXCVIII

2. Given the following values, write the corresponding Roman numerals.

a) 8

b) 23

c) 45

d) 102

e) 319

f) 477

g) 816

h) 1393

i) 1575

j) 1993

ANSWERS FOR PRACTICE PROBLEMS

SECTION I

1) Write each of the following ratios in fraction form and solve for the Unknown X:

a) $\dfrac{50 \text{ mg}}{1 \text{ tablet}} = \dfrac{X \text{ mg}}{5 \text{ tablets}}$ X mg = 250 mg

b) $\dfrac{100 \text{ mg}}{1 \text{ mL}} = \dfrac{400 \text{ mg}}{X \text{ mL}}$ X mL = 4 mL

c) $\dfrac{X \text{ grams}}{2 \text{ capsules}} = \dfrac{5 \text{ grams}}{10 \text{ capsules}}$

X grams = 1 gram

d) $\dfrac{25 \text{ mg}}{X \text{ cc}} = \dfrac{300 \text{ mg}}{480 \text{ cc}}$ X cc = 40 cc

e) $\dfrac{\$1.00}{2 \text{ tabs}} = \dfrac{\$X}{16 \text{ tabs}}$ \$X = \$8.00

f) $\dfrac{10 \text{ gtt}}{2.5 \text{ mL}} = \dfrac{240 \text{ gtt}}{X \text{ mL}}$ X mL = 60

SECTION II

1. For each of the following Fahrenheit values, convert to Celsius (Centigrade):

  a) 60° F = 15.6° C

  b) 90° F = 32.2° C

  c) 104° F = 40° C

  d) 108° F = 42.2° C

2. For each of the following Celsius (Centigrade) values, convert to Fahrenheit:

a) 35° C = 95° F

b) 42° C = 107.6° F

c) 22° C = 71.6° F

d) 30° C = 86° F

SECTION III

1. Given the following Roman numerals, write the value for each:

a) XII   = 10 + 1 + 1 = 12

b) XXV   = 10 + 10 + 5 = 25

c) XLVII   = (50 − 10) + 5 + 1 + 1 = 47

d) LXIV   = 50 + 10 + (5 − 1) = 64

e) XCIII   = (100 − 10) + 1 + 1 + 1 = 93

f) CXXIX = 100 + 10 + 10 + (10 − 1) = 129

g) CCCXXXIV = 100 + 100 + 100 + 10 + 10 + 10 + (5 − 1) = 334

h) MCCXXXVII = 1000 + 100 + 100 + 10 + 10 + 10 + 5 + 1 + 1 = 1237

i) MCMXXXV = 1000 + (1000 − 100)+
10 + 10 + 10 + 5 = 1935

j) MCMXCVIII = 1000 + (1000 − 100)
+ (100 − 10) + 5 + 1 + 1 + 1 = 1998

2. Given the following values, write the corresponding Roman numerals:

a) 8   =   VIII

b) 23   =   XXIII

c) 45   =   XLV

d) 102   =   CII

e) 319   =   CCCXIX

f) 477   =   CDLXXVII

g) 816   =   DCCCXVI

h) 1393 =   MCCCXCIII

i) 1575 =   MDLXXV

j) 1993 =   MCMXCIII

CHAPTER 10 PROBLEMS

1) Write each of the following ratios in fraction form and solve for the Unknown X:

a) 250 mg : 1 tablet : : X mg : 3 tablets

b) 200 mg : 1 mL : : 4800 mg : X mL

c) X grams : 12 capsules : : 5 grams : 24 capsules

d) 125 mg : X cc : : 7500 mg : 480 cc

e) $1.75 : 7 tablets : : $X : 46 tablets

f) 20 gtt : 12.5 mL : : X gtt : 150 mL

2) For each of the following Fahrenheit values, convert to Celsius (Centigrade):

a) 42° F

b) 101.5° F

c) 99° F

d) 128° F

3) For each of the following Celsius (Centigrade) values, convert to Fahrenheit:

a) 37° C

b) 40.5° C

c) 26.4° C

d) 32° C

4) Given the following Roman numerals, write the value for each Roman numeral, solve the problem, then write the solution to the problem in Roman numerals:

a) XIII + CXV =

b) XV + XLII =

c) XCV – XXIV =

d) CXIV – XLIX =

e) DCXIII + CDXIII =

f) XCIX + CI + LXXIV =

g) MMCCCXXVI – MCMXIX =

h) MLII – DI =

5) The medical record on the patient states that this patient had a temperature of 38° C. Today the temperature is 100.9° F on your thermometer. Is this an increase, decrease, or same as yesterday?

6) The surgical procedures require the patient to remain hypothermic (low body temperature) at 80° F for the entire procedure. Unfortunately the patient monitoring

system only reads out values in Celsius. At what temperature in Celsius (Centigrade) does this patient need to be maintained?